BREAST CANCER

PSYCHO-SOCIAL ASPECTS OF EARLY DETECTION AND TREATMENT

For T. – who coped

BREAST CANCER

PSYCHO-SOCIAL ASPECTS OF EARLY DETECTION AND TREATMENT

A Workshop Meeting Report

Edited by P. C. Brand
and P. A. van Keep

The International Health Foundation

MTP

Published by

MTP Press Limited
St Leonard's House
St Leonardgate
LANCASTER

ISBN 978-94-010-9138-1   ISBN 978-94-010-9136-7 (eBook)
DOI 10.1007/978-94-010-9136-7

Contents

List of Participants   vii

Preface   ix

1   'Reach to Recovery': *C.M.*   1
    Discussion

2   Women who have had a mastectomy need increased psycho-social support. How do these women value mutual support groups? *J. M. Wenderlein*   9
    Discussion

3   Mastectomy — experiences of women and professional helpers: *C. M. van Brederode*   15
    Discussion

4   Couples and mastectomy: *E. Metze*   25
    Discussion

5   Adjustment to mastectomy: the psychological impact of disfigurement: *C. Ray*   33
    Discussion

6   Psychiatric problems after mastectomy: *G. P. Maguire*   47
    Discussion

7   Delay in seeking medical advice for breast symptoms: *M. Humphrey*   57
    Discussion

8   Reconstruction of the breast — some considerations: *J. Baruch*   67
    Discussion

CONTENTS

9   Psychological problems related to the
conservative treatment of breast cancer:
P. Juret   73

Discussion

10   Psychological reactions of breast cancer
patients to radiotherapy: *K. Gyllensköld*   81

Discussion

11   Factors affecting participation in cancer
screening programmes: *L. Vermost*   91

Discussion

12   Participants and non-participants in a
mammography mass screening – who is
who: *W. J. A. van den Heuvel*   97

Discussion

General Discussion   105

Index   113

List of Participants

President:
Dr P. A. VAN KEEP,
International Health Foundation,
Geneva, Switzerland

Chairman:
Dr P. C. BRAND,
International Health Foundation,
Geneva, Switzerland

Participants:
Professor J. BARUCH,
Plastic Surgeon,
Centre Hospitalo-Universitaire Henri
    Mondor,
Faculté de Médecine,
Paris XII, France

Dr C. M. VAN BREDERODE,
Social-Psychologist,
Nederlands Instituut voor Sociaal
    Sexuologisch Onderzoek,
Zeist, The Netherlands

Dr K. GYLLENSKÖLD,
Psychologist,
Department of Education,
University of Stockholm,
Stockholm, Sweden

Dr W. J. A. VAN DEN HEUVEL,
Psychologist,
Studiecentrum Sociale Oncologie,
Amsterdam, The Netherlands

Dr M. HUMPHREY,
Psychologist,
Department of Psychology,
St George's Hospital Medical School,
London, England

Dr P. JURET,
Oncological Endocrinologist,
Centre Régional François Baclesse,
Caen, France

C.M.,
Volunteer Worker,
'Vivre comme Avant' (French equivalent
    of 'Reach to Recovery'),
Paris, France

Dr G. P. MAGUIRE,
Psychiatrist,
The University Hospital of South
    Manchester,
Manchester, England

Dr E. METZE,
Psychologist,
Danish Cancer Society,
Ega, Denmark

Dr C. RAY,
Psychologist,
University College,
Cardiff, Wales,
United Kingdom

Dr L. VERMOST,
Sociologist,
Department Sociologie,
Afdeling Medische Sociologie,
Katholieke Universiteit Leuven,
Louvain, Belgium

Dr J. M. WENDERLEIN,
Gynaecologist–Psychologist,
Frauenklinik mit Poliklinik und
    Hebammenschule der Universität
    Erlangen-Nürnberg,
Erlangen, West Germany

Preface

Undoubtedly, the medical aspects of mammary carcinoma – its cause, early detection and treatment – have received considerable attention. Rightly so. The disease is widespread and may be regarded as one of the most important health hazards for women.

The psycho-social aspects of the problem, however, have so far received far less attention. Yet these aspects are of the utmost importance, as became evident once more during our workshop conference, of which this book presents the proceedings. It dealt with two aspects of psycho-social problems resulting from breast cancer:

1. The psycho-social difficulties that women may face when the diagnosis is given and when mastectomy has been performed.
2. The psycho-social factors that play a role in participation or non-participation in screening programmes for mammary carcinoma.

These two areas, and some related topics, have been the subject of a 2-day meeting in Brussels, organized by the International Health Foundation. A number of papers was presented and discussed. The meeting ended with a general discussion.

The editors are grateful to the participants for their willingness to share their knowledge and ideas with them. It is hoped that this book will be of some help to all those who are involved in the treatment and the care of women who are to undergo or who have had a mastectomy and to those who plan the strategy of screening programmes for carcinoma of the breast.

Patrick C. Brand
Pieter A. van Keep

1
Reach to Recovery

C.M.* (Paris)

No woman can imagine what it is like to awake from anaesthesia to discover that one of her breasts is gone, to find only bandages where a breast has been. It is such a traumatic experience that scars remain – forever on her body, sometimes for as long in her mind.

To lose a leg or an arm is certainly a more severe handicap in daily life, but the woman who loses a breast feels, understandably, that she has lost an essential part of her female identity; it has been an assault on her feminity and is experienced as nothing less than a calamity.

It must be almost impossible for a man to understand the extent of the trauma that a mastectomy means for a woman and it must be equally very difficult to understand for a woman who has not had a mastectomy. Yet help and emotional support in the early days after mastectomy may prevent serious problems later. It is this support that is given by a programme such as 'Reach to Recovery'.

A woman said, 'I had a mastectomy 3 years ago; I am not yet cured here'. At the word 'here' she did not point with her finger at her chest, but at her head!

THE PROGRAMME

'Reach to Recovery'† is a programme to supply practical and psychological support to women who have just undergone mastectomy. To accomplish this R.R. uses volunteers, women who themselves have successfully overcome the physical and psychological consequences of the operation.

Briefly, the system works like this: a volunteer visits the woman in the

---

* C.M. are the initials of a R.R. volunteer, whose complete name is withheld at her request.
† In France, the name of the programme is 'Vivre comme avant' (living as before).

hospital 3–6 days after breast surgery. The volunteer answers questions and, simply by being there, serves as an example. Because the volunteer is well-adapted and in good health she reassures the patient. She is like the illustration which conveys more information than a thousand words.

More and more doctors and nurses, who have been convinced of the positive effects of our work, invite R.R. to visit patients before surgery as well as after. We welcome this because the preoperative visit has the same purpose and, hopefully, the same effect as the postoperative one. We tell the patient that we will be back a few days after her operation to answer further questions. We hope that R.R. will gradually become a place of refuge where women can turn for help with all non-medical problems which follow a mastectomy.

The programme has proved itself in the USA, where over 8000 volunteers, all former mastectomy patients, visit 57% of all recently operated women in hospital. In France we now visit 50 to 75 mastectomy patients per week. I myself have visited nearly 300 patients in the last 18 months.

THE VOLUNTEERS

It is obvious that selection of volunteers for the programme is of paramount importance. The selection is also extremely difficult. The surgeon should be sure that the volunteers, whom he allows to talk freely to his patients, are carefully chosen, well-trained and capable of coping with the problems that may arise.

Originally, only women who had had a mastectomy were trained as volunteers, but now women who have had a tumourectomy, or received chemotherapy or radiotherapy also receive training.

We are satisfied if, out of every ten women who offer themselves as volunteers, one or two are found to be healthy and stable enough to meet our standards.

Three times a year all volunteers meet to evaluate their experiences and to improve their methods to help others.

THE VISIT

The rules of the programme lay down that:

A volunteer never visits a patient without the permission of the surgeon in charge.

A volunteer never discusses any medical questions.

Total secrecy between patient and volunteer is guaranteed.

On her first visit the volunteer offers the mastectomy patient a gift of a temporary prosthesis, made of Dacron, lightweight and washable. Although this gift may seem trivial, it is a significant one; it is essential for the patient's morale, because this gift will enable her to leave the hospital with a normal silhouette, as this type of prosthesis can be used immediately.

The patient also receives a pamphlet with all the relevant information to help her to resolve her particular problems. She is also given a little ball which she can immediately use in her physical rehabilitation programme.

Each patient is visited only once in the hospital but the volunteer leaves her name and telephone number, so that the patient can contact her if she has further questions or if she simply wants to talk to someone who understands her reactions which may seem so paradoxical to those around her.

THE EXPERIENCE

The purpose of the programme is certainly not to systematically collect data. If I report here on my experience as a volunteer this presentation must be seen as a summing up of many – certainly not all – facets of my experience.

There are all sorts of reactions after mastectomy and no woman can predict her own. These women are not simply statistics, they are wives, mothers, sisters, daughters, friends and mistresses and there are subtle variations in each case. Not all women who undergo a mastectomy will have psychological problems, but no one can judge in advance who will have them and who will not. It seems therefore wise to offer the possibility of support to all.

Knowledge does not replace experience. Even nurses, who have a vast experience in helping mastectomy patients, sometimes underestimate the need for the support that R.R. can offer. These nurses sometimes doubt whether it is necessary to visit older patients. Age, however, is no guarantee for the absence of problems. A patient 85 years of age: 'I knew you were visiting patients like me in the hospital, but I thought that you might have considered me to be too old. Though mastectomy may be an ordeal, morally and aesthetically, for young people, for us older women it is an added problem for an old body that is already suffering. It is too much to bear.'

The word 'cancer' stands, in the minds of patients for the worst possible illness and having cancer makes the patient aware of the chance of dying. The breasts are in a woman's mind a symbol of womanhood and the loss of a breast makes the patient afraid of having to live with a mutilated body. Again here, age has little to do with the severity of the problems.

A patient of 91 years told me, crying, 'It is so sad for my husband. Please help me with my silhouette'. Her husband was 94. I discovered that in her cupboard she had a curly, white wig which she used during the visiting hours in the afternoon.

It is wise to explain to recently operated patients that they will have periods of depression and that it is good for them to cry. Patients will accept depression without panic if they understand that it is normal to mourn over the

3

loss of a part of their body. Patients are told that they should have confidence in those around them that they love: their husbands, children and friends, because they will help them.

Obese people sometimes have difficulty in accepting their own bodies after having lost – willingly and deliberately – much weight. Imagine the distress then, of a woman who loses her breast, against her will, because of necessity, her breast being a visible, tangible part of herself, a symbol of her femininity and she has to adapt, almost overnight, to a radical change in her body image.

There are no magic words that can solve everything, but the volunteer, from her own experience, can identify herself with the mastectomy patient. The patient senses this and will speak more freely about her anguish, her fears of no longer being a woman, to a person who knows what she is going through and understands how she feels.

A patient said: 'I want to ask you something personal, something very intimate'. The question surely could only have been answered by someone who had experienced the same situation.

THE MESSAGE

A woman should not let her mastectomy become the focal point of her life. Unfortunately, if she is not helped to adapt, she may make the rest of her life pivot around her operation.

A woman, operated on 4 years earlier, said to her husband during a quarrel: 'How dare you speak to me in a tone like that. I have had a mastectomy'.

Patients must be helped to reconstruct an image of themselves that is worthy of being loved, worthy of still enjoying the good things of life. The patient is told to dress as elegantly as possible, to make the most of this, to be at her best. She must become aware that even with only one breast, she has the duty and right to live like other people. Women sometimes think that a mastectomy will change really everything.

A woman, several days after the operation, said: 'And I, who loved art and music so much . . .'

Life is more important than a good figure and a breast amputation sometimes induces women to rearrange the order of their priorities in life.

A woman of about 50, fashion designer in Paris, said 3 months after surgery: 'To me what has happened to my breast is unimportant in comparison with what I discovered in hospital; the moral values of everyone, of doctors, nurses and other patients. I had no idea of this and told my husband that what I learned during those days of my operation is more gratifying than to produce the most beautiful collection.'

R.R. tries to help each woman in her search for her own resources and

4

to help the woman to accept responsibility for her own adjustment to having to live with a single breast.

THE RESTRICTIONS

A volunteer can never leave the hospital under the assumption that the patient she has just seen has accepted her mastectomy, because having to adjust is a time-consuming process. At best, every day will bring her a little closer to acceptance. The volunteer can only point out the positive aspects that remain and, through offering herself as an example, show that by adapting to her mastectomy, a woman can become more understanding, more complete and even more feminine in the true sense of the word.

The volunteer must remember that she will not always be accepted, and that she too is restricted in her struggle against social customs. The volunteer must be careful and must sense quickly what should be said and done and, even more so, what should not be said and done.

The volunteer's possibilities are restricted by the fact that she is dealing with a patient who is horizontal and vulnerable, whereas she herself is upright and in control. She must always walk, figuratively, on tiptoes and then she, as well as the patient, will discover that 'a visit is a sharing'.

Discussion

Wenderlein: What percentage of all women who undergo a mastectomy in France are seen by your organization?

C.M.: We would of course like to visit all women or at least all women whom doctors and nurses think might benefit from such a visit. The programme, however, started only about 2 years ago. We see nowadays about 60 women per week, but I do not know what this means as a percentage of all cases of mastectomy.

Wenderlein: If the decision to invite you is left to the nurses are you then not dependent on their views? Not all nurses may be such good psychologists that they know when to call you and when this is not necessary.

C.M.: You are right, nevertheless we think that the nurses must be involved in deciding who will be visited and who will not. I must say that things gradually become easier for the volunteers when they have had more contact with a particular nurse. Before a patient is seen the volunteer contacts the nurse to ask about the patient's age, mood and other details that can help her prepare for seeing this patient.

van Keep: Who sponsors your organization financially?

C.M.: Reach to Recovery is sponsored and financed by the Cancer Society of each country in which the programme is accepted.

Ray: I would be interested to know what the long-term beneficial effects of such visits are. In the hospital environment women sometimes feel very secure and believe that they will be able to adjust to the mastectomy because of the support they are receiving at that time from doctors, nurses and other patients, and of course from volunteers such as yourself. Once they return home, the picture changes.

C.M.: We do not know the long-term beneficial effect, but we do try to be also of help after the patient has left the hospital. The pamphlet that each patient receives from me gives my telephone number and she can telephone me daily between 8 and 9. We cannot contact them ourselves because we do not ask for the patient's address. We only have the addresses of those who have specifically asked us to remain in contact with them.

Baruch: What percentage of the women you visited have contacted you later, for example during the first year after surgery?

C.M.: About 10%.

Baruch: Would you conclude from this, that only 10% have problems?

C.M.: Certainly not. The reason why women contact me depends on many factors and not only on the presence or absence of problems.

Maguire: Although I am very sympathetic to the use of volunteers, I know that many surgeons in the United Kingdom are hesitant to call on volunteers. They have doubts about the volunteer's selection and training. Could you tell us more about this?

C.M.: A volunteer is never chosen and trained shortly after she was treated herself. We believe that she should have learned to cope with her own problems. Generally that requires a year and a half. Special attention is paid in the selection of volunteers as to their stability, their ability to communicate and their tactfulness.

Training is, apart from learning some basic rules, done 'on the job'. I was invited by Mrs Timothy, who originated the programme in France, to accompany her at visits. I came only to listen and watch in order to learn. After each visit, we discussed the conversation to help me understand the patient's attitudes and reactions.

Then I had to visit the patients myself, but with Mrs Timothy being present. That was, believe me, not at all easy: no more words of advice and explanation, but only a human being in front of me: the patient with all her anxieties.

This period was followed by a long period of time in which I made visits in a hospital where another trained volunteer was also working so that we could turn to each other for advice. Then I was considered as being able to work independently. Later I was asked to assist in the training of new volunteers.

The whole training period is also a period of screening. I think that our programme and our individual performance improve constantly. We learn from each visit and all volunteers meet regularly to share their knowledge. We help – and are happy to be able to help – women who go through a difficult period. We, in Reach to Recovery, work with what we call in France 'Le Coeur à l'Ouvrage'; we work with our hearts and I think that this is why we succeed in helping.

2
Women who have had a Mastectomy need Increased Psycho-social Support

How do these women value mutual-support groups?

J. M. WENDERLEIN

The psycho-social adjustment required from a mastectomy patient is an integral part of her rehabilitation process. Failure to realize this is often due to the fact that even in large centres for the treatment of malignant disease there are not enough physicians and social workers who have received sufficient psychological training. For that reason the psycho-social treatment of the psycho-physical trauma of a mastectomy is often not as good as it could be, or the complex learning process which is associated with it sometimes lasts a very long period of time. In either case the patient is left with a considerable mental burden. Would mastectomy patients be helped by regular meetings from a psycho-social point of view? The successes of an organization which has set itself similar objectives for the support of colostomy patients tend to support that view. At the regular meetings of the association, practical questions concerning ileostomy or colostomy are discussed, but the psycho-social aspects also receive attention. Another example of a self-help organization in which psycho-social rehabilitation is the prime objective is 'Alcoholics Anonymous'. Organizations providing mutual aid for mastectomy patients are found supraregionally in the USA (Reach to Recovery) and in France (Vivre comme Avant).

No such organization exists in the Federal Republic of Germany at present. Would help provided by such an institution be appreciated by German women? The answer to this question was given within the framework of a study of screening procedures for carcinoma of the breast in which 533 women completed a questionnaire. One of its objectives was to determine which type of woman would expect the greatest benefit, while another aim of this pilot investigation was to obtain a first indication of the psycho-social disadvantages compared with the advantages of such an organization.

RESULTS AND DISCUSSION

To the question 'Do you think that regular meetings of women who have had a mastectomy would be helpful?' the following replies were given:

> −yes, definitely   20%
> −yes, probably   52%
> −no   28%

The answers to this question showed no relationship with age, marital status, parity, standard of education or intelligence of the women concerned. Consequently these factors could not be used to provide a first selection for the formation of self-help groups of mastectomy patients, which in the remainder of this text will be referred to as mastectomy groups.

Personality factors

It was found that emotionally labile women regard mastectomy groups as helpful twice as often as emotionally stable women (according to the FPI-N*) ($p < 0.05$).

This is a first indication of the significance of psychological personality factors in the formation of such groups.

In order to avoid mutual reinforcement of anxiety and insecurity, the psycho-social dynamics in these groups should be determined by the emotionally stable woman. As these women are in the minority, they must be well-versed in the basic laws of group dynamics to be able to accomplish this. This applies particularly to the fears resulting from a mastectomy.

Emotionally stable women with a mastectomy should be trained for that responsibility by physicians and social workers, perhaps during the after-care they receive following their operation. In addition other prerequisites must be fulfilled. These women should have coped adequately with the diagnosis of mammary carcinoma and they should be prepared to help other women, in the same circumstances as themselves, to deal with their psycho-social problems. This implies that it would not be sensible to leave mastectomy patients who hold regular meetings to themselves. At least in the beginning, especially selected mastectomy patients with positive group experiences or trained staff members of a clinic or an institution should control the group dynamic processes and correct them whenever necessary.

---

* FPI-N = Freiburg Personality Inventory with 12 sub-tests.

This is not further elaborated upon here because it seems that theoretical considerations could be more usefully linked to the first practical experiences with mastectomy groups.

Attitudes to health care

The more important women considered screening procedures for the prevention of breast cancer to be, the more often they thought that regular meetings of mastectomy patients would be very helpful ($p < 0.01$). This could mean that within such groups one would mostly encounter patients with a relatively good prognosis. Their expectations and problems would be different from those women who have a bad prognosis due to a later recognition of the presence of mammary carcinoma. The problems of early diagnosis and the difficulties encountered in giving advice on the prognosis will not be discussed here.

Women who relied on self-examination for the detection of small superficially located nodules in the breast were particularly convinced that the meeting of mastectomy patients would be helpful ($p < 0.05$). This result of the pilot study also tends to indicate that women with early detected mammary carcinoma would be mostly interested in such groups. When they were asked how long after the discovery of a non-painful nodule in the breast they would wait before seeing a doctor, one-quarter of the women interviewed admitted that they would wait for more than a week. The women in this group expected least benefit from regular meetings of mastectomy patients ($p < 0.05$). Women who said that they thought often about cancer attached more importance to and expected more help from regular meetings of mastectomy patients ($p < 0.01$) than those who did not.

Mastectomy as a psycho-social burden

One-third of all women thought that a period of more than 3 months would be needed for the process of recovery and this indicates that mastectomy has severe psycho-social implications. In the case of hysterectomy only one in every ten women questioned thought that a period of more than 3 months was needed for recovery. The longer the necessary recovery period was estimated to be the greater was the value attributed to mastectomy groups ($p < 0.01$). For women who have recently had a mastectomy it will be helpful to learn from others who had their mastectomy longer ago how much time they needed to learn how to cope after their operation. This applies to almost all areas of the patient's life: to her relationships with her partner or husband and her friends, to her leisure time and working activities. One-half of the women interviewed expected difficulties in their relationship with their partners as a result of the mastectomy. These women were twice as often in favour of regular meetings of mastectomy patients as the women who did not expect any psycho-social problems to arise in their relationship with their partners ($p < 0.01$). Similar results were encountered with regard to the feeling of self-sufficiency after mastectomy. One-half of the women interviewed had lost that feeling and would therefore expect psycho-social help from the mastectomy group.

Women in mastectomy groups will certainly discuss problems concerning their sexual relations. This follows among other things from the fact that women who regarded their breast as extremely important – as did half of all women questioned – were also particularly convinced that regular mastectomy meetings would be useful ($p < 0.05$).

The question of knowing to what extent the partner should or could take part in these meetings can only be answered after practical experience with such groups has been obtained. Many other questions remain which can only be answered by a supraregional organization which should arrange regular meetings of mastectomy patients and design plans for prospective studies. To that effect it would be necessary to collect psycho-social data right from the beginning in a systematic manner and to document the patterns of behaviour in the various groups. This should be done in such a way that the advantages and disadvantages of such groups could be evaluated and compared methodically and statistically. It would be hard to justify the existence of a supraregional organization of mastectomy groups without knowledge of its consequences. Under no circumstances should this concept lead to a greater popularization of group therapy as it is practised today, that is almost as a fashion under different psychotherapeutic guises and in most cases without any substantial scientific control of its results.

Gynaecologists will need to obtain the advice of clinical psychologists, pedagogues and sociologists. In the last instance, however, they will have to assume responsibility themselves for the psycho-social rehabilitation of their patients within the framework of such mastectomy groups as part of the total medical follow-up of patients with malignant disease.

SUMMARY

Is recovery from the psycho-social aspects of the trauma caused by mastectomy made easier by regular meetings of these patients? What kind of women expect most help from such meetings? Initial information is provided by a study of 533 women. Seven out of ten women expected benefit from regular meetings and this proportion was not affected by age, marital status, number of children, level of education or level of intelligence. Twice as many emotionally labile women expected help from mastectomy groups as emotionally stable women.

The more importance women attached to screening for cancer ($p < 0.01$)

the more confident they were of being able to discover breast nodules themselves through self examination ($p < 0.05$), the less they postponed the visit to their physicians for his opinion ($p < 0.05$) and the more often they thought of malignant disease ($p < 0.01$), the more they considered that regular meetings of mastectomy patients would be useful.

The more of a handicap a woman considered the mastectomy to be, the longer the period of time she considered necessary for convalescence ($p < 0.01$), the greater the fear of a deterioration both in her relationship with her partner and in her sense of self-sufficiency as a result of the mastectomy ($p < 0.05$), the more support she expected to receive from such mastectomy meetings.

The results have been discussed with regard to the formation of a supraregional organization of self-help groups.

Discussion

van den Heuvel: I have a question concerning your sample. I understood that they were all patients from the out-patient department, but does this group include women who came because they had breast discomfort or had felt a nodule?

Wenderlein: Patients who came for any complaint related to their breasts were excluded from the study.

van den Heuvel: How reliable do you think that their answers were?

Wenderlein: I am not too pessimistic about that. In our experience there is a good correlation between what women expect will happen and what they experience when the event takes place. Women who expect childbirth to be painful, experience more pain during the event.

van Keep: The crucial question in your interview concerned the usefulness of group meetings of mastectomy patients. This requires women to imagine themselves in a situation which is still rather hypothetical to them.

Wenderlein: This particular question was asked at the end of a long interview lasting about half an hour which dealt with many other problems concerning the breasts. I believe that at the end of the interview women were able to give an answer which reflected their attitudes.

Maguire: What people say they will do in a hypothetical situation may not correlate with how they handle the real situation. You might have obtained more reliable answers if you had interviewed women who had had a mastectomy.

Wenderlein: I have pointed out that our investigation was a pilot study, but I know, from our other investigations, that there may be a surprising correlation between expectation and behaviour. We asked women before the operation how a hysterectomy would affect their relations with their husbands and their sexual behaviour in general. We repeated these questions half a year after the operation and found a surprising similarity in attitudes before and after the event had taken place.

Maguire: You may be right as far as attitudes are concerned. However, it may not hold for the willingness of a given individual to accept help. Nevertheless, what you have said about the use of groups is valuable and interesting.

3
Mastectomy: Experiences of Women and Professional Helpers

Report of a research project

C. M. van BREDERODE

BACKGROUND AND ORGANIZATION OF THE PROJECT

The initiative for this project was taken by NISSO (Netherlands Institute for Social-Sexological Research). The research of NISSO mostly concerns sex experience and relationships in which sexuality is an important aspect. This project was selected because NISSO is becoming increasingly interested in body experience and the body's significance in interrelationships and sex experiences. Its aim was to explore the effects of mastectomy on a woman's body experience, sex experience, self-esteem and on her relationships. The aim also was to collect insights which would contribute to a more systematic care of the patient with regard to psychological and social problems that arise from a mastectomy.

This research was carried out together with Miriam Floor, who is a sociologist. To ensure the relevance of the study design and the applicability of the results, an advisory committee was formed which consisted of people who deal in their daily work with women who had a mastectomy, i.e. doctors, hospital and district nurses and social workers. This committee advised on the project from its start to the final report, which is written for both mastectomy patients and their professional helpers and which will be published in August 1977.

METHOD

We approached women who had personal experience of a mastectomy and also professional helpers, assuming that the latter would give us supplementary information.

We hoped that listening to both women and professional helpers would throw some light on the interaction between them.

We interviewed 30 women about a year after they had a breast amputated. Their ages varied between 30 and 73, they were married or had a partner, they were single, divorced or widowed. They lived in big cities, small towns and in the country, and had been treated in small and large hospitals. Most of them had received radiotherapy after the operation.

The interviews had the characteristics of depth interviews. We started with open questions on a number of themes, followed by more specific questions. Themes of the interviews were:

- experiences in the different periods around the mastectomy:
  - the period between the discovery of a suspicious lump in the breast and admission to hospital;
  - the period in hospital;
  - the period of radiation therapy (this was sometimes started during hospitalization);
  - the period at home after leaving hospital.

Subjects raised for all these periods were the experiences in these specific periods, the need to talk about the loss of a breast at the time, the possibility of talking about it with people in one's own environment such as husband, family and friends and with professional helpers and finally, when this applied, the experience of talking about feelings and worries to others:

- changes in:
- body experience;
- sex experience;
- relationship with partner;
- relationship with children;
- experience of possible contacts with other women who had a mastectomy.

To obtain information from professional helpers we organized group interviews. Thus we had two groups of general practitioners and a group of district and hospital nurses, a group of social workers and a group of radiotherapy technicians. As it was not possible to organize group interviews with specialists, we had individual interviews with two surgeons and a radiologist. All these groups were homogeneous with regard to the professions. Themes of the group interviews were the experiences and the specific problems of the participants in their own work with women who needed a mastectomy, the information they thought should be given to these women and when and by whom this should be done.

RESULTS

Both the women concerned and the professional helpers we interviewed felt that a breast amputation was a very serious change in a woman's life. A breast amputation confronts a woman with two kinds of problems: those problems related to the realization that one has a serious disease, breast cancer, which makes the fear of pain and death more real, and those problems related to the mutilation resulting from the removal of a part of the body that means much to a woman, that reacts sensitively to how she feels, and where many emotions find their expression sexually, erotically and when feeding or cuddling a baby.

Although there is an increase in openness on problems of cancer and death, there is also still a large taboo on these matters and both women and their helpers therefore often have to cope with the above-mentioned problems in surroundings in which there is a tendency to avoid discussing these subjects.

From our interviews it became obvious that a woman does not only require medico-technical help when she has to undergo a breast amputation, but that she also needs at least a trustful relationship with those who give her this medico-technical help. Often she needs specific help with the psychological and social problems that arise from this change in her life.

It is usually relatively easy for a woman to find access to medico-technical help but it is very often not easy to obtain help for her psychological and social problems. This kind of help is not only far more difficult to come by but is frequently even denied to these women. This denial takes the form of belittlement of their problems, of encouraging them to be brave, of stressing that this happens to so many others, or of offering a prosthesis as the solution for all their problems.

POSTPONEMENT OF INFORMATION

It seems that the medical and nursing professions believe that it is important that a woman should be fully informed about the treatment she has to undergo, but that providing this information is often postponed as long as possible and that it is often not sufficiently specific and detailed. Some examples may illustrate this.

In the period before admission to hospital, when it is not at all certain yet whether the lump in the breast is malignant, there seems to be a tendency not to want to cause what is called 'unnecessary worry'. This reaction is also shown in a woman's personal environment. This attitude can make it impossible for a woman to express her feelings and to receive support for her worries and it may even cause feelings of guilt and inadequacy because she 'worries unnecessarily'. It does not make much sense to think in terms of 'unnecessary worry'. Before it is certain that a tumour is not malignant, a woman has good reasons to worry and to imagine what may happen to her

17

and how that might influence her life. Those women in our group who had realized before the operation that they might well lose a breast and who had given vent to their feelings of fear, revolt and sadness, mentioned how this had helped them in coping with their situation afterwards. It is therefore desirable that the facts about breast cancer – not only the prospect of a complete cure, but also what the treatment involves – are made better known to the public at large. It is also important that these facts should be discussed with every woman who needs to undergo further investigations because of a lump in her breast, even though in only one out of 15 cases the presence of breast lumps result in a mastectomy.

The women we interviewed were in most cases told before the operation about the possibility of a breast amputation. Sometimes they had already realized this themselves before they had heard it from their doctor. But some women said they had not believed that this would really happen to them until they discovered that their breast had been removed when they had recovered from their anaesthetic. Not one of the women in our group had been told beforehand that the operation can also involve the removal of lymph glands and chest muscles and that this can result in a partially handicapped arm. When they heard or discovered this after the operation it caused an additional shock. Many women said how important they thought it was to know about this beforehand.

The fact that radiotherapy may be necessary following the operation is also never mentioned beforehand. Again, this means a new setback at a time when a woman just starts to feel that she is now recovering from the operation. It is even harder when, what the surgeon euphemistically calls 'a couple of radiation sessions', turns out to be 20 sessions or even more. The side-effects of radiation therapy, which can be very annoying, particularly when a large number of sessions is necessary, are again only mentioned just before they present themselves or even later after they have occurred. A possible explanation of why the giving of information is postponed, even if its importance is realized and increased frankness is considered valuable, is that help given by the medical and nursing professions is still synonymous with solving problems and offering a cure. It is difficult to be frank when this cannot be offered with certainty.

What these women told us, however, indicates that they do not expect that kind of help for their problems. Realization of their situation and appreciation of their problems, even if these are only expressed by small signs of understanding such as a word, a gesture or a look, make a deep impression and give great support.

BACK HOME

Coming home is described by these women as both a wonderful and a difficult experience. They discover that there are still things worth living for, they experience love, kindness, practical help from husbands, partners, children and close friends. However, they meet also with forced attitudes – 'nice that you are back again, nothing has changed really' – or aloofness and fear from some people in their close or more remote surroundings which sometimes results in a lasting loss of contact.

Most of the women in our group received no after-care of any type whatsoever. Often the general practitioner or the district nurse came once to ask how things were. In particular the interest of the general practitioner was much appreciated and it was also mentioned as being hurtful and strange if neither he nor anyone else ever came to see them and if the question of psychosocial help never arose during the whole process around the mastectomy.

BODY EXPERIENCE

The experience of the mutilation is dramatically described by some women: 'it is like a bomb crater', 'terrible to look at', 'a rotten feeling under the shower or in front of the mirror', 'it feels so ugly and flat, like a boy', 'it is strange, it makes you another being', 'the asymmetry disturbs me so'. Others feel the change of their body not so intensely, but more than one woman said: 'I know losing a leg is much worse, but this too is such a horrible feeling'.

CONTACTS WITH OTHER MASTECTOMY PATIENTS

Most women, both those with and those without a partner, feel that a man cannot understand what it means to have lost a breast. Some have the same feelings with regard to other women who have not themselves undergone a mastectomy. Those women who had been in contact with others who had had a mastectomy experienced this as a great help. These contacts were mostly incidental, but two women were members of a small 'talking group', consisting of women who had all had a mastectomy. They experienced these contacts as very helpful indeed, providing a support that they did not think they could possibly have obtained from other sources. The other women in our group saw many advantages in organizing contact between women who share the experience of a breast amputation, even if they did not think they would like to participate themselves. They were also aware of the dangers involved such as projecting one's own problems on the others, comparing and competing with one another and mismanaging the difficult situation which arises when someone is doing badly. Mutual aid of women who had a mastectomy is still not often organized in Holland. In one or two hospitals a start has been made with visits to mastectomy patients some days after their operation by women who share this experience and who can tell them about the possibilities of prostheses and who can give other practical advice. From the experiences and the opinions of women in our study the help that those women can give to each other, organized perhaps in such a way that professional help can be called upon if difficulties arise, seems to be a rich and as yet little explored source of support.

PARTNER RELATIONSHIP

In the relationship with the partner the loss of a breast was experienced as an important event which was difficult to handle. There had been a definite change, a change that had hurt both the woman and her partner, for their own as well as for each other's sake. It could make a woman and a man realize how much they meant to each other, how much they needed each other. This could bring them closer together and also improve their sex lives. But most women found the sexual aspects of their relationship more difficult. Some said that they only made love for their husband's sake and that they were very unhappy themselves. Sometimes this feeling passed with time but sometimes, especially in older couples, intercourse stopped completely.

CONCLUSIONS

From the results of this exploratory study the following important requirements to enable a woman to cope with a breast amputation can be formulated thus:

–Information on what might happen to the patient with regard to the operation and possible after-treatment should be sufficient and clear. It is easier for a woman to accept the operation and follow-up treatment if she is given the chance to realize beforehand what may happen and if she has given her previous consent. Women differ to a great extent in what they want to know, in how much they want to know and in the amount of detail they want to know. Those who treat them should therefore not only tell them what *they* themselves think is necessary and sufficient but should make certain of this by asking the women whether the information given is also sufficient for *them*.

–The specific problems caused by a breast amputation should be recognized and accepted and the patient should be informed where she can find help for these problems if she needs it and what the limits are to the help which her surroundings can offer.

–There are differences in the willingness and ability of the professional helpers to provide support with psychological and social problems. This applies to differences between the professions but there are also differences between the members of the same profession. This is inevitable and not very serious, provided there is good coordination between all the helpers who are dealing with the same patient. Each professional helper should also make it clear to the patient what his own limits are and be able to suggest additional sources of support if needed.

Discussion

Ray: Do you make a distinction between what women were actually told by the surgeons and what they remembered being told?

van Brederode: No, because this was not possible in this study. The professional helpers we interviewed were not the ones who were dealing with the patients we interviewed.

The experience of professional helpers is that a large part of the information that is given to the patient is lost. Their explanation is that the patient simply rejects those parts of the information that she does not want to hear. We have the impression that the explanation is a different one, that the conditions under which the information is given may be the reason that so much of it is not really received or accepted by the patient. If the patient had been informed in an atmosphere of trust, in which a good relationship between the helper and the patient could develop and in which the patient could express her feelings better, then the patient would be more receptive.

Baruch: There is for me always a limit to what I can tell the patient. This limit is determined by the many questions that the doctor himself cannot answer before the operation. How radical does the operation have to be? Will radiotherapy be necessary? Will there be lymphoedema? How can I, with all those uncertainties, inform all the patients in detail?

van Brederode: Some surgeons told us this too, but I find this difficult to accept. It must be possible to tell the patient what can happen to her and what the uncertainties are.

van den Heuvel: Are some surgeons not hiding themselves behind these arguments about uncertainties to be able to explain why they have not spoken to the patient, whereas the real reason was that they were afraid of their own emotions? Why can't you mention all possibilities to the patient and all the consequences of each? Then the patient can decide what she wants to hear and what she does not want to hear. When, even for in your opinion valid reasons, you do not tell her, you yourself determine the criteria and not the person who is most concerned: the patient herself.

Baruch: If I have to explain the whole range of possibilities, from the best to the worst, I might unnecessarily frighten the patients. I would have to show them pictures or slides. I am sure that a number of patients, if a mastectomy is indicated, will refuse to be operated on and will turn to those specialists, who, on non-scientific grounds, give conservative treatment only. That is a responsibility that I would rather not take.

Wenderlein: Our experience, not with breast cancer but with other types of cancer, is that over 80% of all patients wanted to be fully informed before the operation. Interviews done 3, 6 and 12 months after the operation showed that the same percentage was still of the opinion that such information was needed before the operation. Those who had been given full information beforehand had perhaps a more difficult time before the operation, but eventually their recovery to a psychological equilibrium was faster.

Maguire: A completely different point: you mentioned that women who had a mastectomy benefited from meeting women who had been through the same experience. Unfortunately, we have found that such contact between patients may sometimes be harmful, for example, one woman had to disconnect her telephone because another mastectomy patient could not stop pouring out her troubles. Maybe there has to be some control over this kind of conttact.

4
Couples and Mastectomy

E. METZE

MASTECTOMY AS A FAMILY PROBLEM

A useful approach when working with cancer patients is to see the problem as a family problem. The therapist is not confronted with a sick and scared patient but with a sick and scared family. The whole family is seriously affected, and especially in the case of cancer of a woman's breast the husband will be even more affected than the other members of the family.

It is necessary to follow this particular approach if one wants to help a patient with the psycho-social problems which inevitably present themselves when the diagnosis of breast cancer has been made. Her husband and her children represent potential resources for help and support to the patient when she leaves the hospital, but their ability to give her this support and help depends on the means of communication within the family.

The therapeutic model used is mainly based on the theory developed by Satir (Satir, 1967) and Manocchio (Manocchio and Petitt, 1976). The basic idea is that by improving communication within the family, one can improve the family's ability to cope with a crisis. It is also possible to recognize beforehand which couples or families will probably develop difficulties later on when somebody in the family becomes seriously ill.

Couples and families have rather fixed patterns of communication. For example the ways in which crises are handled, i.e. the mechanisms which are set into motion, are rather repetitive. One particular family, for example, has been using silence as its way to handle crises. The woman who had twice had a mastectomy, had subsequently accepted a night job, while her husband worked during the day. They only spent time together during the weekends, but then they always had visitors. They have been unable to communicate their feelings without being very hostile to each other. They have been using this pattern during the 20 years of their marriage. What is

25

making it difficult for them now is that, before the wife had had her mastectomies, they had a very active sex life, which served as a safety valve for the expression of their feelings towards each other. The wife finds it difficult to accept that she has physically changed; she has little self-esteem and feels useless and unattractive. More often than not she refuses to have intercourse with her husband when he wants it. They are still caught within their usual pattern, but they can no longer use their former 'safety valve' to express their feelings.

The form and the contents of communication used by a couple reveals, to the trained observer, the nature of their relationship and tells him whether this relationship is sound or not.

MASTECTOMY MEANS CANCER

Breast cancer is an illness which is feared for at least two reasons. Firstly, it is a *cancer*, with all that this implies, and admittedly one with a relatively bad prognosis.

Secondly, it implies the necessity of mutilating surgery on a most important part of the woman's body.

The second aspect has, in general, been mostly noted in the past, but it would be wrong to underestimate the importance of the first one, which implies a threat to the woman's life.

The two most important problems which the patient has to face after surgery are the general fear that the cancer will re-occur and the considerable lowering of her morale because of feelings of loss of femininity and of disfigurement. Her identity as a woman is badly shaken because of the symbolic meaning she attaches to her breasts. The staff of the hospital where the patient receives her treatment can already forestall the development of many problems by making certain observations. It may be possible for them to learn about the patient's fantasies and expectations, to get an impression of the circumstances in which she lives and of how the patient's family copes with the situation.

It is very important to realize that every patient experiences illness in her own unique way. As Caleb Parry has written: 'It is much more important to know what sort of patient has a disease than what sort of disease he has' (from Brythe, 1976).

It may be possible to find out from the husband what his feelings are about his wife's disease and her operation. One should always talk to both the patient and her relatives when they are informed of the diagnosis, the treatment involved and the prognosis. It has great advantages to talk with the couple right from the start, because already early on one will have some insight into the way in which they handle the crisis, into how they support each other, and into the openness of their communication.

It is very important to talk to the patient about the possible loss of her breast before the operation. As pointed out by Schoenberg (Schoenberg *et al.*, 1970), the loss of part of the body can be experienced as the loss of a person. It may prevent problems occurring later on if the patient has been given the opportunity to start beforehand with 'anticipated grieving'.

After the operation the patient must be informed about the findings and about their implications. The fact that she has been found to have cancer should normally never be hidden from her. In Denmark patients are mostly told in a direct manner, although there are of course many different ways of telling them. Unfortunately, many doctors still try to hide from their patients that cancer has been found and tell them, for example, that their breasts have been removed prophylactically in order to avoid the risk that the lesion might later develop into cancer. It is important, however, to impress on the patient right from the start that it is wrong to be afraid to use the word cancer. If the clinician who gives the diagnosis and discusses its implications with the patient is not able to use this word in an open and frank manner, then the patient cannot be expected to do this herself later on. By hesitating to use – or even completely avoiding – the word cancer, the ground is prepared for difficulties which may arise later on for the patient in her relations with husband and family. The person who provides the first information defines the scope of the communication, and if he gives vague information on the nature of the illness then this will make it more difficult for the patient to be able to cope with the illness herself. There is then also the possibility that all communication around the patient will stop and there is a risk that a so-called 'psychosemantic illness' will ensue.

THE HUSBAND'S CONFRONTATION

One of the first problems which faces the couple when the patient has been discharged from hospital, is the husband's confrontation with the inevitable fact that his wife has lost her breast – that she is 'different'. The situation at this point is crucial, because if the husband is not very supportive and understanding at that particular moment a classic 'vicious circle' may develop.

It is difficult for most women to cope with this situation, because they themselves have not yet accepted their mastectomy and they feel ashamed and have very little self-confidence, while they also fear that they are going to be rejected because of their mutilation.

The couple can be helped to overcome this critical phase if it is discussed with them in hospital before it arises, with both the patient and her husband present. They should be encouraged to both face this problem as soon as possible. A very common reaction from these women is to instruct their husbands not to look at them and to hide in the bathroom while they undress.

The feelings these women have about themselves are projected onto the husbands, then these women blame them for their reactions. This is the classic 'vicious circle' which is a very common occurrence. The husbands, of course, are often very anxious in this situation and when they show their anxiety, the suspicions of their wives are reinforced. Once this chain of reactions has started, the main purpose of therapeutic intervention must be to explain this process to the couple. This is done by means of a cross-interview technique, where the partners are encouraged to express their feelings about each other and to tell each other about their fantasies around the situation. It can even be necessary that the therapist very explicitly provokes a confrontation; this can be rather dramatic but also be very helpful.

THE SEXUAL RELATIONSHIP

To re-establish sexual relationships is another important step towards normalization. If the confrontation which was described above has been coped with, and if both partners have more or less accepted the change, there should be no serious problems in this respect. If the communication has not been re-established properly, a very common problem may arise (which is certainly not exclusively seen in the couple where the wife has had a mastectomy), namely that the patient regards the attempt to re-establish a normal sexual relationship as a gesture of politeness and not as a genuine desire from the husband. There too therapeutic help and guidance may be required. This can be a fairly long process, depending on how the woman is able to re-establish her feeling of self-esteem. If the husband understands this process and realizes what is going on in his wife, then he can also support and reassure her, for example, by the manner in which he makes his advances to her.

MASTECTOMY AS A CRISIS

As mentioned before, mastectomy must be seen as a kind of crisis and as a continuing *process*. It is important not to label the patient at a certain stage as a psychiatric case because she reacts with a depression. The risk of this would be that the patient will become fixed in the role of a psychiatric patient, with all the resulting implications. Of course there will be patients with severe problems and depressions who do need psychiatric help and psychotropic drugs, but depressions have to be seen as normal reactions in women who have had a mastectomy. This is part of their passage through the crisis. This process can be fairly long. Gyllensköld (1976), described women who, 2 years after their mastectomy, have still not been able to emerge from the reaction phase of their crisis.

Depression and loss are clearly linked together. The same can be said about low self-esteem and depression. Bard and Sutherland (1955) have shown that there is a positive correlation between women with a low self-esteem and the severity of depressive reactions following radical mastectomy.

It is very important that the mastectomy patient receives support from her family while undergoing this process. Unfortunately, many couples run into difficulties when one of them is depressed, mainly because they react by applying the common-sense principle that the way to cure a depression is to pretend that it is not there or, alternatively, to pretend that there is no reason to be depressed. As Weakland (1974) has pointed out, if people in contact with a depressed person try to make him feel better by telling him that he should be happy, that he has no reason to feel depressed or that he is not allowed to be depressed, they will probably, instead of helping him, perpetuate his state of depression. What started originally as a sadness has thus become a depression. When passing through a crisis after a mastectomy it is important to accept the woman's depression and grief, and to establish a communication with her which allows for this fact that the patient feels sad. This enables her to show her feelings of depression and provides her with proper support during this process. The therapist should emphasize this when he counsels the family.

MASTECTOMY AND THE CHILDREN

Unfortunately it is not uncommon that parents try to hide from the children that their mother has had a mastectomy. In terms of communication they create a secret in the family. This kind of consideration is very destructive to relationships within the family. Even small children sense that something is happening. The result is that various forms of disturbed behaviour appear in these children such as enuresis, school phobia and even delinquency. The therapist should be aware of this possibility and, if necessary, organize a therapeutic session with the whole family together to help the couple to disclose the secret to their children.

A very common mechanism which may especially occur in families who live in a very closed system of communication, is being so considerate to each other that Laing's famous description of games would be appropriate: 'They are playing a game. They are playing that they are not playing a game . . .' (Laing, 1972). If it goes on for a long time, then this kind of consideration for each other is very destructive to family life, because it blocks the possibility of growth within the family. This mechanism should not be confused with the 'denial charade', which is a way of dealing with serious problems in which both parties are very open about what they are doing, and in which both are in agreement.

THE COUNSELLOR

Who should be the counsellor? This is to a certain extent dependent on both cultural and structural factors. In Denmark the physician traditionally acts as counsellor for patients with psycho-social problems and sometimes the social worker does. There are no organized facilities for the counselling of cancer patients. Most doctors do not have time to deal with the emotional problems of their patients. Moreover, most doctors give this kind of work a very low priority. Finally, they are rarely trained to counsel. It is difficult for physicians, who have almost exclusively been trained in the natural as opposed to the behavioural sciences, to deal adequately with the severe emotional problems that occur in cancer patients. It is very difficult for the physicians to switch from the physical nature of disease to its emotional aspects. Neither the patient nor her relatives expect from the physician that he deals with the emotional aspects. In many cases they even try to adapt their communication with the physician to the biophysical framework that he prefers, or more correctly, the framework that they think he prefers. This, of course, is an interaction between two parties in which it is difficult to say who is putting whom in what role.

Another important problem in the relationship between physician and patient is that of dependency. Most patients try to act as good patients, which means that they try to avoid behaviour which they think will upset the physician. They do not want to be considered troublesome patients who bother the physician with their emotional problems. It may be difficult, however, to establish a satisfactory relationship between physician and patients as far as help in the psycho-social area is concerned. The best solution will be the use of a team approach, in which physician, nurse, 'Reach to Recovery' volunteer and a person who is trained in psychotherapy, together treat the patient and her family.

It is difficult to estimate how many couples and families are in need of psycho-social therapy. Doctors and nurses in the oncological wards estimate that one-third of their patients need this sort of therapeutic help. If a team approach is used, it will be possible to identify psycho-social problems at an early stage and to start preventive therapy before new ones can develop.

CONCLUSION

The psycho-social problems which the mastectomy patient and her family have to face are of great importance. Several authors have pointed out that open communication, sharing of feelings and support for the patient within the family seem to be important factors in connection with survival times and rates of relapse. (Carlson, 1975; Seligman, 1975; Bahnson, 1975). Further research in this field is required. Rehabilitation on the psycho-social level is therefore just as important as physical rehabilitation.

References

Bahnson, C. B. (1975). Psychological and emotional issues in cancer: The psycho-therapeutic care of the cancer patient. *In: Seminars in Oncology*, Vol. 2, no. 4

Bard, M. and Sutherland, A. M. (1955). Psychological impact of cancer and its treatment. IV: Adaption to radical mastectomy. *In: Cancer*, **8**, p. 656

Quotation from: Blythe, P. (1976). Stress. (London: Pan Books)

Gyllensköld, K. (1976). Visst blir man rädd . . . (Lund: Forum)

Laing, R. (1972). Knuder (English edition: *Knots*). (København: Rhodos)

Manocchio, T. and Petitt, W. (1976). Families under stress. (London: Routledge & Keagan Paul)

Satir, V. (1967). Conjoint family therapy. (Palo Alto: Science and Behavior books)

Schoenberg, B., Carr, A. C., Peretz, D. and Kutscher, A. H. (Ed.) (1970). *Loss and Grief: Psychological Management in Medical Practice*. (New York: Columbia University Press)

See f. ex. Carlson, R. (ed.) (1975). *The Frontiers of Science and Medicine*. (Chapter 3) (London: Wildwood House)

Seligman, M. E. P. (1975). *Helplessness: On Depression, Development and Death*. (San Francisco: Freeman)

Watzlawick, P., Weakland, J. and Fisch, P. (1974). *Change*. (New York: Norton Co.)

Discussion

van Brederode: How do husbands react to your suggestion to discuss problems that may arise later?

Metze: In general the husbands react in a positive way, more than two-thirds of those who are invited accept.

van Brederode: It is an often heard complaint that hospital wards do not offer the chance of any privacy for the couple, such as a room where they can be together without being seen and heard by other patients and by the staff.

Metze: You are right. Some hospitals, however, do have such facilities. I regard these as very beneficial.

van Keep: Have you, in your counselling, ever noticed that women change the way in which they talk about their breasts? It struck me that women who normally spoke about 'my uterus', suddenly changed to '*the* uterus' after they had been informed that a hysterectomy was needed, as if an organ that has become a threat to their existence no longer has the right to be part of them.

Metze: Although I never registered this consciously, I have noticed that women suddenly speak of *the* breast, after they have been given the diagnosis.

Ray: Do you try and guide couples towards a particular strategy after the mastectomy or do you vary your guidance depending on the couple's own means of defence? I could imagine that, whereas for one couple silence could be the solution, for another this might not be so. The woman might like to take a dependent role and the husband a caring role, while other couples might like to joke about the situation.

Metze: There is certainly no particular strategy which applies to all couples. I try to find out how the couple has handled crises before and, if this was done adequately, whether this same strategy can also be used for the mastectomy.

van den Heuvel: Did you discover in that way any characteristics of the couples which indicate whether they will need help?

Metze: I am concentrating on the ways in which the partners are dealing with each other, how they communicate and how they share their feelings. At present it seems to me that in particular those couples are at risk who have difficulties with the sharing of feelings. I hope, in the future, to be able to give more detailed advice on this to nurses so that they will be able to recognize these patients.

5
Adjustment to Mastectomy
The psychological impact of disfigurement

C. RAY

The breast is not an organ of great functional importance, particularly within those age groups most vulnerable to breast cancer. It might on these grounds be argued that its loss should be relatively easy to accept, and that mastectomy should involve fewer difficulties of adjustment than many other mutilative surgical procedures. Indeed, in one study women were asked to what extent they would miss various parts of their body if these were removed, and their responses indicated that they would rather lose a breast than their tongue, their nose, an eye, a foot, an arm or a hand (Weinstein *et al.*, 1964). Nevertheless, the breast does have a symbolic significance which is independent of any physical function which it performs: its loss may threaten a woman's self image and it may do so in two different ways. Firstly it may challenge the integrity of her body image, making her feel mutilated and thus 'stigmatized'; secondly it may challenge her identity as a woman, making her feel less attractive and less able to act out a feminine role. The aim of the study to be described in this paper was to assess the longer-term impact of the loss of the breast upon a small, randomly selected, sample of patients. Since the emphasis was upon reactions in the longer term, adjustment was assessed at an interval of 18 months to 5 years after surgery. It was hoped that by this time the patients' attitudes would have become relatively stable: that they would have encountered all the personal and social difficulties associated with the loss of the breast and have learned to cope with these to the best of their ability. The subjects in the sample selected for this study had all had a simple or modified radical mastectomy; they were at that time free from any sign of recurrence, and their ages ranged from 39 to 63.

Adjustment to the operation was assessed from two different perspectives.

33

Firstly the mastectomy sample was compared with a control group of cholecystectomy patients on a number of standard psychological measures; these included measures of depression and anxiety, together with various measures relating to self-image.* It was predicted that the women who had had a mastectomy would be more depressed and anxious, and more negative in their self-image, than those who had had a cholecystectomy. This sort

Table 5.1 Mean adjustment scores for the two surgical groups (*n* = 30 pairs)

	Mastectomy	Cholecystectomy	t value	p
Depression	42.0	33.7	1.85	<0.05
Anxiety	42.6	36.0	1.83	<0.05
*Self-esteem	2.1	1.5	1.62	NS
*Social warmth	13.9	14.4	−0.56	NS
*Social abrasiveness	34.2	32.3	−1.58	NS
*Social attractiveness	28.5	27.6	0.74	NS
*Introversion–extraversion	23.6	27.3	2.10	<0.05
*Body cathexis	39.5	42.6	−1.55	NS

* Inverted scale
NS = not significant

of approach produces data which allow for a comparison between the two surgical groups in terms of their *general* attitudes toward life and toward themselves. It does not, however, yield more specific information about the mastectomy patients' current attitudes toward their operation and its implications: it is these attitudes which would, presumably account for any general differences observed between these subjects and the control group. The data obtained from the psychometric approach, employing standard psychological measures was thus supplemented by data obtained within an interview setting. Here the mastectomy patient's feelings about the operation were the specific focus of concern, rather than her general psychological adjustment. These two approaches were not kept completely separate, and an attempt was made to relate some of the information obtained during the interview to subjects' scores on the measures of depression, anxiety and self-image.

Firstly, let us look at the comparison of the two surgical groups (Table 5.1). Significant differences occurred on three of the measures employed: depression, anxiety and introversion, with the mastectomy patients being more anxious and depressed, and more introverted in their behaviour. Note that the introversion–extraversion scale referred to is not the EPI; the measure used in this study required subjects to rate themselves on a number of adjectives associated with behaviour in a social setting, and a score in an introverted direction here reflects a self-description characterized by social

* Costello and Comrey, 1967; Rosenberg, 1965; Veldman and Parker, 1970; Secord and Jourard, 1953.

withdrawal and passivity. In addition to the above differences the mastectomy group tended to be lower in self-esteem than the control group, and this difference closely approached significance ($p = 0.06$). The three scales of social warmth, abrasiveness and attractiveness are similar to the introversion scale in that they are based upon subjects' self ratings on adjectives relevant to social attitudes and behaviour. The absence of significant differences between the groups on these scales suggests that the mastectomy subjects did not feel either less warm or more hostile toward others, and did not see themselves as less socially attractive. Nor were they less satisfied with their general physical appearance than the cholecystectomy group ('body cathexis').*

Turning next to the interview material, let us review very briefly the attitudes expressed by the mastectomy subjects toward the loss of the breast. These attitudes were both varied and complex. There was however, one simple distinction which could be made between individuals, and that was in terms of the apparent degree of concern which they currently felt about their disfigurement. Some appeared to be genuinely unconcerned about this, while others claimed that the loss of the breast had had adverse effects upon their feelings about themselves, their sexual relationship with their husbands, and their general poise. These two groups of mastectomy patients were compared on those measures which had discriminated between the mastectomy and cholecystectomy patients (see Table 5.2). Those subjects who

Table 5.2 Mean adjustment scores for subjects expressing high and low concern about disfigurement ($n = 14$, $n = 16$ respectively)

	High concern	Low concern	t value	p
Depression	47.6	35.6	1.78	<0.05
Anxiety	44.9	40.1	0.94	NS
*Self-esteem	2.4	1.7	1.26	NS
*Introversion–extraversion	21.1	26.4	2.64	<0.01

* Inverted scale
NS = not significant

reported an absence of concern were significantly less depressed and less introverted than the other mastectomy subjects; they were also less anxious and had higher self-esteem, but not significantly so. It is interesting that the differences between these two mastectomy groups reflected to a considerable extent the differences observed between the two surgical groups. On each measure the direction of the high concern–low concern difference was the same as that for the mastectomy–cholecystectomy difference, and two of the three comparisons which were statistically significant in the latter case were significant also in the former.

Now the loss of the breast is not the only aspect of mastectomy which may be a source of concern to the patient. The diagnosis of cancer implied by this operation may also produce distress,* and a fear of recurrence was apparent in the responses of many subjects interviewed in the present study. It might be suggested that patients who did and did not admit to anxiety about recurrence might be compared on the general measures of adjustment, as were those patients who differed in their concern about disfigurement and that the relative influence of these two sources of concern might then be determined. It is, however, very difficult to obtain valid accounts of patients' fears for their future health. Some individuals who claim a lack of concern may be behaving defensively and refusing to acknowledge their fears, and there was some suggestion of such defensive behaviour in the interviews carried out in this study. In order to make a valid comparison it would be necessary to carry out a more intensive exploration of this topic, distinguishing those subjects who are genuinely not concerned about the possibility of recurrence from those subjects who are attempting, perhaps unsuccessfully, to defend against anxiety.

The following conclusions may be suggested on the basis of the findings obtained in this study. Firstly, that mastectomy does have an adverse effect upon a woman's attitudes toward life and toward herself; women who have had a mastectomy are more depressed, more anxious and more introverted than an equivalent group of women who have not had this operation, and they tend to be lower in self-esteem. Secondly, that these effects are to some extent associated with the woman's concern about her disfigurement: those women who claimed a lack of concern in this respect were less depressed and less introverted than those who expressed a greater degree of concern, and there was a tendency for the former group to be less anxious and to have higher self-esteem. Lastly, it should be emphasized that there is a high degree of individual variation in adjustment to the disfigurement produced by mastectomy: some women appeared in interview to be relatively unaffected by this, while others still felt considerable grief and resentment about their loss several years after the operation.

References

Bard, M. and Sutherland, A. M. (1955). Psychological impact of cancer and its treatment. IV. Adaptation to radical mastectomy. *Cancer*, **8**, 656

Costello, A. J. and Comrey, A. L. (1967). Scales for measuring depression and anxiety. *J. Psychol.*, **66**, 303

Maguire, P. (1975). The psychological and social consequences of breast cancer. *Nursing Mirror*, 54

Quint, J. C. (1963). The impact of mastectomy. *Am. J. Nursing*, **63**, 88

Renneker, R. and Cutler, M. (1952). Psychological problems of adjustment to cancer of the breast. *J. Am. Med. Assoc.*, **148**, 833

---

* Renneker and Cutler, 1952; Bard and Sutherland, 1955; Quint, 1963; Maguire, 1975.

Rosenberg, M. (1965). *Society and the Adolescent Self Image.* (Princeton: Princeton University Press)

Secord, P. F. and Jourard, S. M. (1953). The appraisal of body cathexis: body cathexis and the self. *J. Consult. Psychol.*, **17**, 343

Veldman, D. J. and Parker, G. V. C. (1970). Adjective rating scales for self description. *Multivariate Behav. Res.*, **5**, 295

Weinstein, S., Sersen, E. A., Fisher, L. and Vetter, R. J. (1964). Preferences for body parts as a function of sex, age and socio-economic status. *Am. J. Psychol.*, **77**, 291

Supplementary notes

SAMPLING PROCEDURE

The subjects in the mastectomy group had all taken part in the Cardiff–St Mary's trial (Forrest *et al.*, 1974). Those patients from the trial who were between the ages of 35 and 65, who had had the operation from between 18 months and 5 years previously, who were currently free from any sign of recurrence, and who had no other serious illness or disability, were considered eligible for this study. An equivalent list of cholecystectomy patients was drawn up, with selection being based upon similar criteria for age, time since surgery and current health, but with the additional criterion that patients described in their records as 'obese' should be omitted from the list. The latter procedure was intended to reduce the expected difference in mean weight between the two surgical groups. The samples were selected from these two subject pools in pairs, each mastectomy subject being matched with a cholecystectomy subject for both age and the interval which had elapsed since surgery. Patients so selected were contacted by letter, and asked whether they would be willing to participate in a project designed to find out how people feel about different operations and how, if at all, these have affected their lives. Where a patient refused, another of similar age and time since surgery was selected from the relevant pool. There were seven refusals from mastectomy patients, and five from cholecystectomy patients. The final samples consisted of 30 subject pairs. Ages in the mastectomy group ranged from 39 to 63 with a mean age of 53.05 years, while the age range of the cholecystectomy group was from 42 to 62 with a mean of 52.75 years. For both groups the mean interval since surgery was 3 years 5 months, with a range of 1 year 8 months to 4 years 11 months for the mastectomy subjects and a range of 1 year 8 months to 5 years 3 months for the cholecystectomy subjects.

INTERPRETATION OF THE COMPARISON BETWEEN SURGICAL GROUPS

Mastectomy was found to be associated with poorer general adjustment on measures of depression, anxiety, introversion and, possibly, self-esteem.

Such an association does not necessarily justify the inference of a causal relationship. It might be argued that the differences observed between the two surgical groups existed prior to surgery, and that the subjects in the mastectomy group would have differed from a control group on these dimensions prior to surgery and prior to the development of their cancer. In other words, women who are *vulnerable* to breast cancer may be more depressed, anxious and introverted than the average woman. This hypothesis, that certain personality types are associated with a predisposition to cancer, is one that has commonly been advanced, but it is difficult to obtain evidence which either clearly supports or refutes the hypothesis. Subjects are usually tested or interviewed after development of their symptoms, diagnosis and treatment, and any differences observed between cancer patients and controls could well be explained as an outcome of these experiences rather than as a pre-illness personality disposition. One of the better controlled studies in this area, and one which deals specifically with breast cancer patients, is that of Greer and Morris (1975). In their study patients with breast symptoms were tested prior to formal diagnosis; those who were later diagnosed as having a cancerous growth were found to differ from those with benign conditions in the expression of emotion, but not in reported levels of depression, neuroticism or extraversion. This suggests that the higher depression, anxiety and extraversion scores of the mastectomy group in the present study are not attributable to personality differences which existed prior to diagnosis and treatment: although the measures employed in the two studies were different, they are conceptually similar. Moreover, it may be noted that studies which have suggested an association between extraversion and breast cancer claim that individuals vulnerable to this disease tend to be dispositionally *extraverted* (Coppen and Metcalf, 1963; Hagnell, 1966). The finding that women who have had a mastectomy describe themselves as being relatively *introverted* in their attitudes and behaviour contrasts strikingly with the above claim. In summary, the inference that the differences observed between the two surgical groups reflects a reaction to surgery does here appear to be justified, and the differences observed between those mastectomy patients who did and did not report concern about the loss of the breast further supports this position.

THE INTERVIEW

All of the subjects were asked to discuss their feelings about their operation, following administration of the tests, but the mastectomy subjects were encouraged to do this in particular detail. Interviews for these subjects ranged from 45 minutes to 2 hours in length and were recorded on tape. Material relevant to the study was later transcribed from each subject's tape onto cards, with different cards being used for material relating to different issues, e.g. husband's reaction. In most cases little prompting was needed in the form of direct questions and the interview was conducted as an informal discussion rather than according to a scheduled format. Several issues were explored in the course of the interview. The subject was firstly asked to describe the experience of mastectomy in retrospect: her feelings when she first discovered the breast abnormality; her reaction on being told of the possibility of mastectomy; the impact of the operation itself; her husband's reaction. Discussion was then directed toward the subject's current attitude toward the operation, particularly with respect to the loss of the breast and the disfigurement which this entailed. While care was taken not to imply that this should lead to difficulties, the subject was asked whether the loss of the breast had had any impact upon her feelings about herself, her relationship with her husband, or any other aspect of her life. She was also encouraged to talk about her attitude toward the diagnosis of cancer and the possibility of recurrence, but only when she herself mentioned these issues. It was suspected that at least a few of the subjects would not have been explicitly informed of their diagnosis, while others may have repressed this information; in such cases any suggestion that their condition may have been a serious one, or that there might be current cause for concern about their health, could have been extremely threatening. Four of the women in the sample did not themselves refer to the health implications of the mastectomy, and no conclusions may be drawn about their attitudes. Even where the subject did refer to this aspect of the operation, it was not always possible to probe too deeply into the attitudes which she expressed because of a danger of challenging defences which served to reduce anxiety. The data obtained from many of the subjects on this topic must thus be regarded as incomplete.

CONCERN ABOUT THE LOSS OF THE BREAST

The low concern group

Fourteen of the women interviewed claimed that the loss of the breast had had little impact upon their lives. The breast for them appeared to have little psychological significance and they reacted to its loss as they would to that of any non-functioning body part. They were able to camouflage their disfigurement with the help of a prosthesis, and this was for them all that was required. Some were able to imagine that women other than themselves might be concerned, and suggested that they too might have experienced such concern in different circumstances: if their husband had reacted negatively, if they had been younger, if they had a larger bust, etc. For the majority of this group no adjustment to this aspect of the operation was required, and they were able to accept the loss of the breast without difficulty.

The high concern group

The 16 women in this group expressed feelings of sadness and bitterness about their disfigurement. They claimed that they no longer felt fully women, although such feelings were often only salient when they were depressed about things in general. Some were secretive about their mastectomy, even to the extent of avoiding people who had found out about this. Others were also self-conscious about their operation, but attempted to cope with their embarrassment by being deliberately open and direct about the fact that they had had a breast removed; a few even joked in public about their disfigurement, again to reduce the feelings of social constraint experienced by either themselves or those with whom they were interacting. These women *were* distressed by the loss of the breast but they were anxious not to let others see this, and anxious that their social image should not suffer. Many of the women in this group disliked the sight of themselves when undressed, and avoided looking at the scar. Those who were married tended to be modest about their nakedness in front of their husbands, and about half of these women claimed that their sexual relationship had suffered as a result of the mastectomy. None of the latter felt that their husband's affection or sexual desire had decreased; they all admitted that it was their own feelings which had changed. Two of the subjects had refused sex since the operation and were considerably distressed about the impact which this had had upon their relationship. Three of the women in this group were without a husband at the time of the interview, and these felt that their chance of marriage or remarriage, or of any other relationship with a man, had been destroyed because of the loss of the breast.

CONCERN ABOUT CANCER

Fifteen of the women with whom this was discussed admitted to experiencing some anxiety about the possibility of recurrence. For a few of these this was a constant threat. They monitored their health and attempted to lower the risk by such precautions as sleeping and eating well; many were careful to protect their other breast from knocks, the belief that breast cancer may be caused by a blow being commonly voiced. Most of these 15 women, however, made a deliberate attempt to put the possibility of recurrence from their minds, having decided not to live their lives in the shadow of this threat. They were fully aware that the cancer might recur, but saw no point in anticipating something which might not in fact happen. These women could not, however, avoid all anxiety. Their fears were awakened whenever they experienced symptoms such as tiredness or headaches for which they had no immediate explanation, and all were rather nervous about the time of their routine check-up at the hospital. The remaining women, 11 in number, claimed that they experienced no anxiety about their health. Three of these were fully aware that the mastectomy had not necessarily 'cured' the disease, but they denied all concern about this, two because they were very distressed about the loss of the breast and saw the threat to their health as being relatively unimportant, and one because of an extremely fatalistic attitude. The other eight women who claimed to experience no anxiety felt this way either because they did not foresee a possibility of recurrence, or because they saw this possibility as remote. They quoted reassurances which they claimed they had been given by the hospital staff; they pointed out that their growth had been extremely small, that they had not delayed before consulting their general practitioner, or that breast cancer is not the same as other cancers in that it is easier to treat.

This sample of 26 may be divided into two groups, according to whether or not concern was expressed about the cancer, and their scores on the measures of general adjustment compared. Such a comparison was in fact made, with the prediction that those subjects who expressed concern would be less well-adjusted and that the differences between these groups would parallel the differences observed between the mastectomy and cholecystectomy groups. No significant differences were, however, found (see Table 5.3).

Table 5.3 Mean adjustment scores for subjects expressing high and low concern about health ($n = 11, n = 15$ respectively)

	High concern	Low concern	t value	p
Depression	42.4	38.1	0.59	NS
Anxiety	40.7	47.5	−1.21	NS
*Self-esteem	·1.7	2.9	−2.12	NS
*Introversion–extraversion	23.3	24.5	0.49	NS

* Inverted scale
NS = not significant

Indeed, the subjects who were apparently more anxious about the possibility of recurrence had *lower* anxiety scores. They were also *higher* in self-esteem, and this difference would have been statistically significant if a difference in this direction had been predicted. It is, however, probably inappropriate to attempt to differentiate between subjects in this simple dichotomous fashion given the complexity of reactions to this aspect of mastectomy. Not only the individual's reaction to the possibility of recurrence must be considered but also her perception of the likelihood of this. Thus there were some subjects who both acknowledged that the cancer might recur and admitted to considerable anxiety in this respect. There were others who were aware of this possibility but tried to avoid thinking about it in order to reduce their anxiety. There were those subjects who did not avoid contemplating the possibility of recurrence but claimed not to experience any anxiety about this. Finally, there were those who claimed not to recognize any significant risk to their future health and thus saw no reason for anxiety. Moreover, we might also consider whether the reactions of the last two groups were or were not defensive, and if they were defensive, whether or not they were successful in eliminating anxiety. A separate study, and methods other than those that might be employed within an interview setting, would be needed to explore these issues.

References

Coppen, A. J. and Metcalfe, M. (1963). Cancer and extraversion. *In:* Kissen, D. M. and LeShan, L. L. (eds.) *Psychosomatic Aspects of Neoplastic Disease.* (London: Pitman Medical)

Forrest, A. P. M., Roberts, M. M., Preece, P., Henk, J. M., Campbell, H., Hughes, L. E., Desai, S. and Hulbert, M. (1974). The Cardiff–St Mary's trial. *Br. J. Surg.*, **61**, 766

Greer, S. and Morris, T. (1975). Psychological attributes of women who develop breast cancer: a controlled study. *J. Psychosomat Res.*, **19**, 147

Hagnell, O. (1966). The premorbid personality of persons who develop cancer in a total population investigated in 1947 and 1957. *Ann. N. Y. Acad. Sci.*, **125**, 846

Discussion

Baruch: Why did you choose cholecystectomy patients as controls? To study the impact of disfigurement resulting from mastectomy it might have been better to compare such patients with those who had a facial disfigurement.

Ray: It would indeed be interesting to compare the relative impact of facial surgery and mastectomy, but the disfigurement involved in these two cases will not be equivalent in degree. Any differences in psychological reaction could be accounted for either by the visibility or the extensiveness of the disfigurement.

Maguire: Have you checked the post-operative diagnoses of the cholecystectomy patients? It is known that neurotic patients sometimes undergo this operation for rather vague symptoms, for example unexplained pain in that area. If there were a number of such patients in your control group that would have minimized the differences you found with the mastectomy group.

Ray: I have not checked the pathological findings. The only effect would have been, as you said, to increase the differences observed.

Wenderlein: I understood that you collected your data a number of years after the operation, but that way you cannot compare the personality before and after the operation.

Ray: I am indeed presuming that the effects that I observed were reactions to the operation; I assume that the differences in personality did not exist before the operation.

van den Heuvel: Were the two groups matched on psychological criteria?

Ray: No, they were matched for age and for the interval between surgery and the interview. There were no social class differences. The only noted difference was that the cholecystectomy patients had a significantly greater body weight, even though I had excluded from the sample patients described as obese in their medical records.

Brand: The greater body weight may have affected body cathexis and social attractiveness.

Ray: This may have affected the data. There was a strong tendency for the cholecystectomy patients to be less satisfied with their general appearance and their figure. They also regarded themselves as less socially attractive. The difference in body weight might perhaps be the reason for my not finding predicted differences on these two scales – social attractiveness and body cathexis – between the mastectomy and cholecystectomy groups.

van den Heuvel: It strikes me that about half the sample expressed low concern and about half expressed high concern. In a recent article of Greer and Morris the percentages were 75 and 25 respectively.

Ray: I think that my criteria of 'high concern' may well differ from those of Greer and Morris; we will have a different subjective threshold between low and high concern. I do not want to claim or imply that half of these women suffered extreme distress after the operation.

Humphrey: Was there any relation between your interview data and the meaning of the breast for the individual women? Did you ask for example about breast feeding, breast sensitivity in lovemaking and the importance of the breast for their body image?

Ray: No, I did not. The interview in some cases lasted for as long as three hours, including administration of the tests, and it was not possible to deal with all relevant points.

Brand: Does marital status influence a woman's reaction to mastectomy?

Ray: Only six of the women were not married and so a statistical comparison was not possible. In terms of the interview responses, the unmarried women seemed if anything more concerned, even when they were over the age of forty, because they felt that the loss of a breast had destroyed their chances of marriage or of any other relationship with a man.

van Brederode: The unmarried women in our sample suffered as much from the loss of a breast as the married women did.

Baruch: Married women and unmarried women do differ in their attitudes towards surgery on the breast – not only for breast reconstruction but also for hypertrophy and hypotrophy. Two-thirds of the women in which I did a breast reconstruction were unmarried. The married women often had marital difficulties.

6
Psychiatric Problems after Mastectomy

P. MAGUIRE

Seventy-five women aged 65 years or less who presented with a breast lump and later had a mastectomy were followed up from the time they first attended hospital until 1 year after operation. The women were interviewed at home on three occasions to assess their psychological and social adjustment; before admission for biopsy, 4 months and 1 year after mastectomy.

These assessments were carried out by trained interviewers. They used a series of 4-point scales (0–3) to rate the frequency and extent of any psychological and social problems experienced by the women over carefully specified periods of time. For example, on the depression scale a score of 0 meant that no depressive symptoms had been evident within a given period while a score of 1 indicated that a few symptoms such as low mood or weeping had been experienced infrequently, with well periods between. When the symptoms of depression had been persistent and occasionally severe enough to include ideas of hopelessness, suicide and worthlessness a score of 2 was given. A score of 3 was reserved for those who experienced even more persistent and severe symptoms of depression including frequent suicidal ideas and plans.

Clinically, a score of 2 meant that the depression was serious enough to require medical help either from a general practitioner or a psychiatrist. A score of 3 indicated the need for more intensive psychiatric help.

A control group of 50 women who presented with breast lumps which were found to be benign (either immediately upon their first attendance or after biopsy) were followed up in an identical way. These control subjects were drawn at random from those who were of similar age, social class and marital status to the women included in the breast cancer group.

The inclusion of this control group made it possible to determine how much any psychiatric problems which were found in the breast cancer group were due to the cancer and its treatments.

ANXIETY BEFORE BREAST BIOPSY

Where the lump had been discovered 6 months or less before attendance at the clinic, ratings were made of the 3-month period before discovery to establish how anxious the women were before they realized that they had any breast trouble. Where they had discovered the lump over 6 months before attendance at the hospital, a period of 3 months before they decided to seek help was taken as the baseline period.

In this way 11% of those women who turned out to have breast cancer and 10% of the benign group were found to have experienced moderately severe or severe symptoms of anxiety in this 3-month baseline period (Figure 6.1).

After discovery of the lump or decision to seek help there was a sharp increase in the percentage of women in the breast cancer (21%) and benign group (26%) who complained of anxiety.

In the benign group there was a clear fall in anxiety levels after they had seen their general practitioners and the surgeon. However, in the group who had breast cancer there was a further increase in the percentage of women with moderately severe or severe anxiety symptoms. Hence by the time of admission for biopsy, 27% of the cancer patients but only 14% of the benign group were experiencing such anxiety.

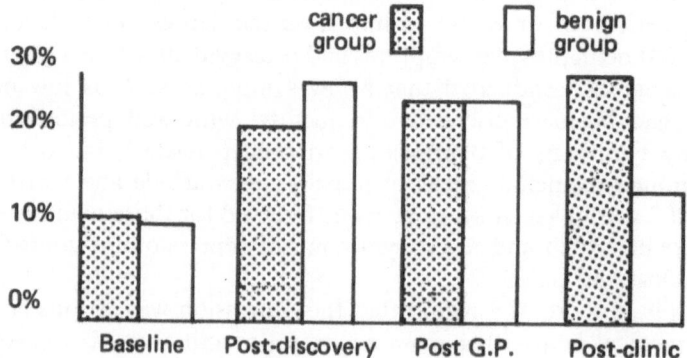

Figure 6.1 Percentage with moderately severe or severe anxiety symptoms

DEPRESSION BEFORE BIOPSY

Five per cent of the cancer group and 12% of the benign group were rated as having moderately severe or severe depression in the baseline period

(Figure 6.2). While there was little change in the benign group in the period leading up to the clinic or biopsy, there was a somewhat more marked increase in the levels of depression in the breast cancer group.

Overall, 31% of those women who were to have a mastectomy were depressed and/or anxious in the pre-biopsy period.

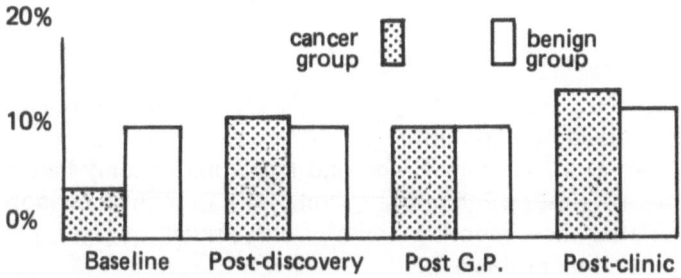

Figure 6.2   Percentage with moderately severe or severe depressive symptoms

REACTIONS AFTER MASTECTOMY

Ratings made at the follow-up interviews which were conducted 4 months after mastectomy revealed a two-fold difference in the incidence of moderately severe or severe depression between the breast cancer and benign groups (Table 6.1).

Table 6.1   Depressive reactions after mastectomy

	4 Months		1 Year	
	Cancer	Benign	Cancer	Benign
None	31	32	31	35
Minor	24	12	28	11
Moderate	19$\Big\}$27%	6$\Big\}$12%	11$\Big\}$21%	4$\Big\}$8%
Severe	1	0	5	0

This difference was still evident 1 year after mastectomy.

Over one in five of the women who had had a mastectomy were found to be suffering from moderately severe or severe depressive symptoms.

Anxiety symptoms were also more prevalent in the mastectomy group both at 4 months and 1 year later (Table 6.2).

In all, 19 of the 75 women (25%) who underwent a mastectomy were suffering from an anxiety state and/or depressive reaction 1 year later.

In contrast, only six of the 50 (12%) benign patients were affected similarly.

The difference in the amount of anxiety and depression noted in the two

49

Table 6.2 **Anxiety reactions after mastectomy**

| | 4 Months | | 1 Year | |
	Cancer	Benign	Cancer	Benign
None	32	34	28	32
Minor	27	12	33	14
Moderate	14 } 21%	4 } 8%	12 } 19%	4 } 8%
Severe	2	0	2	0

groups was even greater when any mood changes which occurred in the study period were taken into account.

Four times as many women who had had a mastectomy had developed a medium-term (lasting 2–8 months), long-term (8 months or more) or late (beginning after the 4-month follow-up – still present at 1 year) anxiety or depressive reaction (Table 6.3).

Table 6.3 **Duration of mood disturbance**

| | Anxiety reactions | | Depressive reactions | |
	Cancer	Benign	Cancer	Benign
None	40	35	36	40
Short term	10	15	13	4
Medium term	9 } 33%	0 } 10%	8 } 35%	2 } 12%
Long term or late	16	5	18	4

Only six of the 19 women in the mastectomy group who were found to have mood disturbance at 1 year had already been anxious or depressed in the baseline period.

SEXUAL PROBLEMS

Many more of the mastectomy group were found to have suffered from sexual problems than the benign group during the follow-up period (Table 6.4). One in three of those women who had had a satisfactory and active sex

Table 6.4 **Sexual problems**

| | Initial interview | | At 4 months | | At 1 year | |
	Cancer	Benign	Cancer	Benign	Cancer	Benign
None	40	26	25	27	26	28
Minor	4	7	4	5	6	5
Moderate	3 } 5%	3 } 8%	6 } 40%	2 } 11%	11 } 33%	1 } 8%
Severe	1	0	13	2	5	2
Not applicable	25	13	25	13	25	13
Not known	2	1	2	1	2	1

life before operation had either ceased to have any sex life or any enjoyment from it 12 months later. Only 8% of the benign group experienced similar problems.

As with mood disturbance, the differences in sexual adjustment over the study period were even more obvious when any upset in sexual adjustment was allowed for. Over half of the mastectomy group (54%) had experienced medium- or longer-term changes (Table 6.5) compared with only 8% of the benign group.

Table 6.5   Duration of sexual problems

	Cancer	Benign
None	21	31
Short term	1	2
Medium term	10 } 54%	0 } 8%
Longer term or late	16	3
Not known	2	1
Not applicable	25	13

Thus, overall, 29 of the 75 (39%) women who had a mastectomy were judged to have developed a longer-term depressive reaction, anxiety state and/or sexual problem within the first year which was serious enough to warrant medical or psychiatric help.

HELP GIVEN

Unfortunately, only eight of the 19 women with anxiety and/or depression at 1 year had been able to give their own general practitioners any real idea of what had been happening to them; and three of these had already been receiving psychiatric treatment from their practitioners in the baseline period. Hence, of the 16 'new cases' only five had mentioned their difficulties directly. A further two women had complained about other problems but been perceived to be in need of psychological help.

The general practitioner's response was to prescribe psychotropic drugs (Table 6.6).

Despite the prevalence of depression either alone or accompanied by anxiety, anxiolytics and hypnotics were given more frequently. Only two of

Table 6.6   Nature of drugs prescribed

Mood Disturbance	Hypnotic	Anti-depressant	Anxiolytic	Not known	Patients
Moderately severe	7	1	3	2	8
Severe	1	1	2	0	2
Total	8	2	5	2	10

the six patients with severe reactions (Table 6.7) received any medication.

Even where the women did get drugs, all but two complained of the lack of any opportunity to discuss their worries.

Table 6.7 Nature of mood disturbance at 1 year

Anxiety	3
Depression	5
Anxiety and depression	11

While the role of drugs and counselling in these reactions still needs to be determined, it is likely that the more severe reactions would have benefited from more appropriate medication, particularly antidepressants.

It was also striking that none of those with sexual problems had sought help. They seemed to view them as the price they had to pay for physical survival.

DISCUSSION

Our findings are similar to those of Greer and his colleagues (Greer *et al.*, 1977). They found that 23% of their mastectomy group were depressed 1 year later while 27% had sexual problems.

This high psychiatric morbidity should not be surprising. For when a woman has a mastectomy she has two formidable problems to overcome. She has to come to terms with the loss of a part of her body that may have been of particular importance to her sense of femininity, self-esteem and confidence. She also has to live with the terrible uncertainty of whether she will become ill again, suffer and die.

Furthermore, it has been claimed that the kind of stresses she is under, namely the threat of loss of life coupled with uncertainty about whether or when that loss may occur, are especially likely to cause psychiatric illness (Brown *et al.*, 1977).

A major question is whether this morbidity could be reduced or prevented by the provision of counselling before and after mastectomy. A trial is, therefore, being carried out to determine this. Women who are admitted for

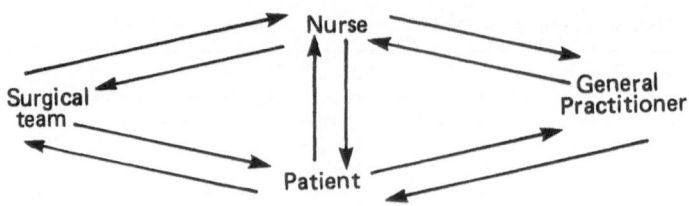

Figure 6.3 Liaison nurse scheme

a mastectomy are being randomly allocated to routine care alone or routine care plus regular visits by a liaison nurse.

The aim of this nurse is to give advice and information about the operation, prostheses and any subsequent treatments. She also monitors their psychological well-being. When problems become evident these are notified to the general practitioner and the surgical team. They are dealt with either by the liaison nurse or appropriate specialist (Figure 6.3).

It is already clear that her monitoring function brings problems to light at a much earlier stage. However, only when the study is completed will it be possible to determine how effective the intervention has been.

References

Brown, G. W., Harris, T. and Copeland, J. R. (1977). Depression and loss. *Br. J. Psychiat.*, **130**, 1

Greer, S. H., Morris, T. and White, P. (1977). Psychological and social adjustment to mastectomy: a two-year follow-up study (to be published)

Discussion

Ray: Do you know to what extent the husbands spontaneously helped their wives to return to a normal sexual relationship?

Maguire: We also studied how husbands reacted to the mastectomy. In general we found that many were too considerate. They would avoid sexual intercourse saying: 'I will leave you alone because you must have had a terrible time'. Their wives interpreted this as 'he does not love me any more'. Communication between the couple may then break down completely.

Brand: Are there social factors, or factors in the patient's medical history, that could help us to predict who might become severely depressed?

Maguire: We found that only six of the 19 women who had mood disturbance had already had problems before their breast trouble. Thus it could not all be blamed on pre-existing psychiatric illness. There were four other women who were depressed before the onset of their breast disease but who coped very well with the mastectomy. Thus psychologically healthy women can become psychiatrically ill as a consequence of mastectomy. This should not be surprising, for mastectomy is the kind of event that precipitates psychiatric illness. It threatens loss but it is uncertain if and when that loss will occur.

Other factors are whether the woman has someone she can turn to, how important her bust is, what previous experience she has had, and social class.

Baruch: I presume that you do not favour reconstruction, but how many women ask for it?

Maguire: In the United Kingdom many surgeons are not in favour of a reconstruction because – among other reasons – there is a risk that recurrences under the prosthesis will not be spotted. There is on the other hand an increasing number of women who ask for some kind of plastic surgery, but I have no idea how often this happens. About one-third of all women are dissatisfied with the external prosthesis they are given and I think that it is in this group that one finds the patients who will ask for reconstruction.

van Keep: Did you study the influence of age on anxiety and depression?

Maguire: There was a tendency for younger women to be more affected, but even women in their sixties were not immune from serious problems. Some women, irrespective of age, do not mind losing a breast providing that they stay alive. Others find the loss of a breast the worst thing that could have happened.

van den Heuvel: What chance is there of curing the one woman out of every five who has such serious problems?

Maguire: While I do not underestimate the problems of accepting such disfigurement, I think most women can, if they are given help, usually come to terms with it. The other major fear – will the cancer come back – can be much more difficult to cope with. Statistical probabilities do not help much. However, in general we seem to be able to help most of those with serious problems. But I am certain that we have not yet found the most effective method of treatment.

van Brederode: I understood from your paper that all women were told what might happen to them, even if this may prove later to have been unnecessary because the lump was benign.

Maguire: The surgeons involved prefer to standardize what they say as much as possible. So they mention the possibility of a mastectomy whenever this is likely to be indicated. They also mention any other treatments such as radiotherapy or chemotherapy. This is done because a randomized trial of different kinds of chemotherapy is being carried out. They therefore must explain this kind of treatment fully in order to obtain informed consent. This often causes upset in the short term but it does prepare these women for what may happen to them. I believe this is a better policy than not telling. A woman who is told about all the possibilities will be relieved if they are not needed. A woman who is not warned that she may need further treatment, will be shattered when she learns that such treatment, for example radiotherapy, is needed.

The results of our present trial will tell us whether this practice is justified or not.

7
Delay in Seeking Medical Advice for Breast Symptoms

M. HUMPHREY

Among malignant diseases breast cancer is the commonest cause of death in women. Recently it has accounted for more than 11 000 deaths annually in England and Wales, 15% of these women being under 50 and therefore likely to have dependent children. It has been estimated that one in every 20 women will suffer from the disorder at some time in her life, and that only one in five of its victims can expect a complete cure (Brinkley and Haybittle, 1968). Not only has breast cancer shown an upward trend of incidence over the years, but there is little evidence of improved methods of treatment. Thus there is plenty to concern the physician and surgeon, and if the medical outlook remains gloomy, it is all the more reason for the social scientist to become interested in the patient's emotional response to a threat of this nature.

When writing on the question of delay in seeking advice about the meaning of early symptoms, I can claim no expertise, merely curiosity on the basis of interviews with 26 women attending a breast clinic early in 1975. At that time I was planning a project on the impact of mastectomy on a woman's self-image, and was not especially interested in the factor of delay. The project was never launched, and on looking through my rather flimsy data I find that only three or four women admitted to having waited longer than three months before seeing a doctor. Since the pioneer study of Pack and Gallo (1938) most authors have taken this period as the criterion for significant delay (e.g. Aitken-Swan and Paterson, 1955; Henderson, 1966; Cameron and Hinton, 1968; Greer, 1974). The patients in my own small study would appear to have acted more promptly than most of those featuring in the literature if my figures are reliable, and I would like to draw attention to the remarkable indifference of all the authors I have consulted to the matter of reliability. Unless the patient's statements are carefully probed they cannot be accepted at face value, and the longer the actual delay the more scope there must be for inaccurate reporting. I can think of one woman who recalled a tingling sensation in her left breast on pulling off her nightie in a hotel bedroom while on holiday. Exactly a week later I saw her at the clinic, and 9 days after that she had a mastectomy. Such a precise diary of events is unusual, and most patients find it hard to pinpoint the onset of a symptom unless it can be linked to an unforgettable event of some kind. If it is reasonable to suppose that many women would hesitate to admit that they had waited a long time before visiting the doctor we may infer that the tendency is to underestimate delay, so that published figures must be regarded as conservative.

There is a further general point to be made before reviewing some of the literature on delay. Underlying the emphasis on immediate consultation is the assumption – or at any rate the hope – that this will improve the prognosis. However, Bloom (1965) in a closely argued paper has pointed out that there is no simple relationship between speed of action by the patient and response to treatment. A crucial factor in treatment is the histology of the tumour, and Bloom found that the more rapidly growing and lethal tumours predominated among women consulting early whereas the less malignant lesions appeared more often in women with a long history. Thus the distribution of histological gradings tends to counterbalance the influence of delay on survival rate. This paradox is not fully explained but could be due to the capacity of highly malignant tumours to produce more alarming symptoms. The author concludes as follows:

'Since almost half the patients with breast cancer who appear to seek treatment early already have axillary metastases, the overall improvement in survival rate resulting from efforts to reduce delay is likely to be limited. On the other hand, since half the patients with this disease attending a cancer hospital in a large city seek advice only when their tumours are greater than 5 cm, or ulcerated, it is difficult to believe that present day methods of treatment are achieving the best possible results. . . . Because of the chance of saving or prolonging useful life for the *individual*, a factor often overlooked in mass statistics, early treatment must be the undoubted principle for all cases of breast cancer' (p. 260).

In the remainder of this short presentation I shall address myself to two questions only: (1) What are the major causes of delay? (2) How can women with breast symptoms be persuaded to act more quickly? My search for answers to the first question has turned up few surprises, but I am still somewhat baffled by the second one.

CAUSES OF DELAY

Among the more commonly cited causes of delay are ignorance, fear of diagnosis, fear of disfigurement from mastectomy, fear of hospitals in general and surgery in particular, and a fatalistic attitude (Greer, 1974). I shall comment on these in turn.

Ignorance has long ceased to be an important factor in delay. Cancer education campaigns have begun to preach the value of regular self-examination of the breasts, and any woman who was motivated to comply with this advice would be almost certain to see her doctor at the first suspicion of trouble. I am not sure whether it is a mark of a healthy, well-adjusted woman to be willing to look for trouble in this way, but it seems unlikely that more than a small minority of women would be capable of acquiring the habit at the present time. Nevertheless there can be few women of normal intelligence who have never heard that a lump in the breast may mean cancer, and therefore calls for urgent medical examination even in the absence of pain as a driving force. It may be partly fortuitous how soon a woman becomes aware of a lump, but the more crucial question is how awareness comes to be translated into action (for sooner or later she will be driven to act). In an early but frequently quoted paper Shands et al. (1951) pointed to the ambiguity of statements about 'knowing', since awareness can occur at many different levels. Thus an individual may know that she has a lump, and that a lump may be a cancer, yet be quite unable to relate the two facts in order to infer that she may have a cancer. Alternatively, she may acknowledge the relationship without feeling constrained to act upon it, just as a neurotic patient may analyse his difficulties with startling clarity but without taking the smallest step towards resolving them (so-called intellectual insight). It is only when new information has been fully integrated with existing knowledge, and allowed to influence personal expectations and behaviour patterns, that true insight can be achieved. In other words, help-seeking in this situation is not a cognitive but an emotional problem, the problem of mastering emotional response to threat.

The next three causes of delay are variations on the theme of fear. Aitken-Swan and Paterson (1959) reported that, of 244 breast cancer patients who had been in touch with a cancer education campaign, a third were too frightened to act on the advice given. The exact nature of this fear will differ from case to case, but fear of the diagnosis of cancer is still commoner that it needs to be because the notion of incurability persists. These authors and others have found that personal familiarity with cancer in a friend or relative, even where the outcome has been satisfactory, is no safeguard against fear of the unknown – indeed, such patients are apparently more prone to delay. Henderson et al. (1958) in a study of 100 cancer patients* in Montreal, 69 of whom took longer than three months to consult a doctor, argued that 'many of the attitudes held by the public – that cancer means inevitable death, that nothing can be done – are often a reflection of the physician's feelings, who hedges over the truth by euphemistic words and

---

* Including 63 with breast cancer.

phrases. These express his own feelings of failure and inadequacy in the presence of malignancy. He consequently avoids frank discussion with the patient in an endeavour to escape from the emotional difficulties that would result in them both' (p. 40). I wish I could confidently assert that this argument had become less valid over the past 20 years, but alas I cannot.

Fear of disfigurement may be a powerful force among patients about to undergo mastectomy, but I have seen no evidence that it deters them from seeking medical advice in the first instance. They are seldom given much time to brood about it in advance and some women have the traumatic experience of waking from the operation without being able to recall any explicit warning of the possibility. (Such was the theme of a moving TV play based on what had happened to the author's wife.) My own experience of mastectomy patients is both limited and superficial, but my impression is that women with sound family support can adapt well to the loss of a breast. The concept of premature death, especially when it may be both painful and lingering, seems to me a far more potent source of anxiety than disfigurement.

Yet it would be mistaken to suggest that a woman's reluctance to present a breast lump for examination is specifically and invariably related to fear of a lethal diagnosis. Some people will avoid consulting a doctor about anything whatever for as long as they can; and if in addition they are averse to contemplating a period in hospital, which may be mentally associated with the need for surgery, one can understand how perception of a lump will lead to procrastination. Once a patient has been admitted for investigation she is unlikely to refuse mastectomy, but awareness of the possibly inexorable sequence of events may deter some women from embarking on the very first step. Even a trusted physician may be helpless in the face of these sort of anxieties, and the fact that he is trusted may tend to keep the patient away rather than bring her forward. It would require a subtle research method to disentangle the components of fear in relation to cancer of any kind, and meanwhile we can but acknowledge the complexity of the problem.

Table 7.1 Distribution of delay at different stages from symptom discovery to hospital admission

Interval	Diagnosis	Degree of delay (months)			
		<1	1–2	3–12	>12
Symptom to GP	Benign	20	1	2	2
	Cancer	30	13	8	5
GP to surgeon	Benign	24	—	1	—
	Cancer	45	2	2	3
Surgeon to hospital	Benign	13	6	6	—
	Cancer	50	1	1	2

N.B. Delay was significantly greater in the malignant group ($n = 57$) than in the benign group ($n = 26$), the proportion consulting a doctor within a week being 25% and 68% respectively ($\chi^2 = 11.05$, $p < 0.001$).
Source: adapted from Cameron and Hinton (1968).

Table 7.2 Patient delay in seeking treatment by diagnosis

Diagnosis	Interval between first symptom and first medical examination (months)				
	<1	1–2	3–12	>12	Total
Benign	67 (74%)	5 (6%)	13 (14%)	5 (6%)	90
Cancer	33 (49%)	12 (18%)	18 (27%)	4 (6%)	67
Total	100 (64%)	17 (11%)	31 (20%)	9 (6%)	157

$\chi^2 = 11.61$, d.f. 3, $p < 0.01$.
Comparing the proportions delaying three months or longer: cancer 33% (22/67); benign 20% (18/90); $z = 1.83$, $0.05 < p < 0.07$.
Source: Greer (1974).

Turning finally to fatalism as a cause of delay, this may be a common deterrent to early consultation in elderly patients. About a third of breast cancer victims are over 70 when they die, and almost two-thirds are over 60. Advancing age may betoken a greater readiness to let events take their course, especially when there are no dependent relatives. In these circumstances it may be reasonable to wait until pain or discomfort are obtruding, and questionable how much pressure should be exerted by friends or neighbours if they happen to be aware of the symptoms. It remains true, of course, that measures designed to improve the *quality* of survival are worth applying, but length of survival may be no longer a paramount consideration.

METHODS OF PERSUASION

Before we can consider how delay in reporting breast symptoms to a physician can be minimized, there is a further curious observation to be taken into account. Both Cameron and Hinton (1968) and Greer (1974) have reported that patients whose tumour turned out to be benign acted more quickly than those whose tumour was subsequently diagnosed as malignant (Tables 7.1 and 7.2). There is no obvious explanation for this paradox, since initial symptoms (with the possible exception of nipple discharge) were not demonstrably different between the two groups. It is almost as if patients with cancer are intuitively aware of their plight, yet feel compelled to defend themselves against this awareness. What can be done to induce a state of appropriate concern in *all* women about their breast symptoms, regardless of ultimate diagnosis?

This is essentially a problem for the psychologist, but in the present state of knowledge I cannot guarantee to offer anything more than a promising lead, and certainly no clear-cut solution.

There is now ample evidence from a series of controlled experiments by various workers over a long period (see, for example, Ley and Spelman, 1967; Rachman and Philips, 1975) that people are more readily influenced by mild propaganda than by strong propaganda when it comes to safeguarding their health or avoiding unnecessary hazards. A threatening message may be later recalled as accurately as a more restrained one, yet in terms of desirable behavioural change the latter is usually more effective. This has been shown in such diverse situations as smoking in relation to lung cancer or dental hygiene in relation to caries. On this basis it is tempting to conclude that cancer education campaigns should stress the probability of a breast tumour being diagnosed as benign, which is in fact close to 80%. Aitken-Swan and Paterson (1959) made this very point, yet after three years of intensive campaigning in a defined geographical area in the North of England the proportion of breast cancer patients who had sought advice within a month of noticing symptoms rose from 28% to no more than 38%. This was surely a disappointing response even granted that there was no gain whatever in a control area without such a campaign.

In the light of this finding, and of my survey of the literature as a whole, I suspect that many women might use any information about the odds in favour of a reassuring diagnosis as a basis for postponing the crucial visit. Those who are unduly anxious about the possibility of cancer would hide behind the defence that they can safely procrastinate while awaiting further developments – if any. I may be wrong and I hope I am wrong, but I am afraid there is going to be no easy way of taking the sting out of cancer without at the same time encouraging a flight into premature optimism. We must seek an escape from the dilemma whereby either we drive potential breast cancer patients away from the medical profession by making them even more apprehensive than they already are, or else we relieve their apprehension before it has even been put to the test.

Let me try to end on a more positive note. I have often been surprised by a woman's ability to conceal a breast lump from her husband, which is perhaps made easier by the declining frequency of sexual intercourse around the time of the menopause when the risk of breast cancer increases. But it is hard to see how a rapidly growing lump could remain concealed for long where the couple made love regularly up to the time of onset, and the normally loving wife who starts to make excuses would surely arouse her husband's suspicions. I appreciate that loss of spontaneity and sexual urgency in the ageing male might serve to create a stalemate, but maybe we can hope to reach these reluctant women through their menfolk. Even if some men are more heavily defended against the threat of cancer than their wives there must be plenty of others who will urge them to take action. In any case a threat of this nature is not something to be faced alone, and although not all marriages are harmonious the great majority in the relevant age group are stable. Future education campaigns would do well to enlist the husband as an ally where he has always set a high premium on his wife's health and happiness, and if members of the audience have ideas on how he might be reached this may be a suitable topic for discussion.

References

Aitken-Swan, J. and Paterson, R. (1955). The cancer patient: delay in seeking advice. *Br. Med. J.*, **1**, 623

Aitken-Swan, J. and Paterson, R. (1959). Assessment of the results of five years of cancer education. *Br. Med. J.*, **1**, 708

Bloom, H. J. G. (1965). The influence of delay on the natural history and prognosis of breast cancer: a study of cases followed for five years to twenty years. *Br. J. Cancer*, **19**, 228

Brinkley, D. and Haybittle, J. L. (1968). A 15-year follow-up study of patients treated for carcinoma of the breast. *Br. J. Radiol.*, **41**, 215

Cameron, A. and Hinton, J. (1968). Delay in seeking treatment for mammary tumours. *Cancer*, **21**, 1121

Greer, S. (1974). Psychological aspects: delay in the treatment of breast cancer. *Proc. R. Soc. Med.*, **67**, 470

Henderson, J. G., Wittkower, E. D. and Lougheed, M. N. (1958). A psychiatric investigation of the delay factor in patient to doctor presentation in cancer. *J. Psychosom. Res.*, **3**, 27

Henderson, J. G. (1966). Denial and repression as factors in the delay of patients with cancer presenting themselves to the physician. *Ann. N.Y. Acad. Sci.*, **125**, 856

Ley, P. and Spelman, M. S. (1967). *Communicating with the Patient.* (London: Staples)

Pack, G. T. and Gallo, J. S. (1938). Culpability for delay in treatment of cancer. *Am. J. Cancer*, **33**, 443

Rachman, S. J. and Philips, C. (1975). *Psychology and Medicine.* (London: Temple-Smith)

Shands, H. C., Finesinger, J. E., Cobb, S. and Abrams, R. D. (1951). Psychological mechanisms in patients with cancer. *Cancer*, **4**, 1159

Discussion

Maguire: We found that 21% of women said that it was their husbands who encouraged them to seek help. So the husband might be the person to concentrate on if we want to shorten the delay. Another 15% said their women-friends had made them go. Perhaps we should therefore look more closely at the influence other people have on the patient with a lump in the breast.

There was also an interesting paradox in how women reacted to particular symptoms. Benign lumps are usually larger, painful and may bleed. Malignant lumps are small and painless. Yet the women regarded larger, painful or discharging lumps as more likely to be cancer. So women with benign lumps sought help earlier.

van Keep: I do not think that health-education campaigns concerning smoking and eating habits can be compared with campaigns for the promotion of adequate behaviour when a lump in the breast has been 'self-diagnosed'. In the second case help-seeking behaviour is advised and I think that many women are confused when on the one hand they are bombarded with stories about overconsumption of medical services to keep them away from the doctor and, on the other hand, with the advice to rush for help when a lump is felt.

Humphrey: There may be conflicting tendencies in health education campaigns, which are each, in terms of content, completely justified. I think that such education should aim at teaching the individual the difference between minor health problems and potentially serious ones, which if Dr Maguire's observations are correct, could be done rather more effectively than in the past so far as breast cancer is concerned.

Wenderlein: Particularly in the lower social strata there are women with limited knowledge about early detection and therapeutic possibilities. These same women think they know enough and they are not motivated to absorb more information.

Humphrey: Most educational campaigns are designed by well-educated, middle-class persons and tend to reach a similar type of person who is less in need of persuasion.

I think, but I may be wrong, that this is not so much of a problem in relation to breast cancer screening as it is in the screening for cervical cancer. In the latter case there is an inverse social class gradient and it seems difficult to reach those who are most at risk. If this is not the case with breast cancer then those designing the campaigns and those who should benefit would be on the same wavelength.

Gyllensköld: In Stockholm a person-to-person campaign was started in which female nurses showed other women how to feel their breasts and told them what to do if a lump was found. In particular it is important to teach them how a lump feels.

Ray: A problem in motivating women to go to their doctor where the slightest doubt exists is that there are only limited incentives: we cannot promise a complete return to health to those women who consult early. It is difficult to phrase our campaigns and to promote the right sort of optimism without misrepresenting the situation.

Humphrey: Even if we did overcome all these barriers and succeeded in having all women self-examining their breasts, then the crucial question would still remain how to induce the patient to seek advice once a lump had been detected. The patient may be quite realistic in thinking that if a malignancy has been diagnosed, she has not actively contributed to improving her own fate. If early diagnosis did make all the difference – as it does in cervical carcinoma – we would be on much firmer ground.

8
Reconstruction of the Breast: Some considerations

J. BARUCH

Plastic surgeons, for many years past, have been paying particular attention to the breasts, which are not only just secondary sex characteristics but also an essential component of female beauty. Because of what they represent to a woman through all phases of her life, removal of a breast is a traumatic event of major proportions. For some women surgical reconstruction may be indicated. But before this is suggested, the surgeon must first of all study the psychological consequences of the mastectomy and then determine if the patient really wants a reconstruction. He must decide why he wants to reconstruct the breast, on whom, and when.

WHY OPERATE?

The first purpose of a reconstruction is to satisfy a patient's wish.

Women who undergo a breast amputation undoubtedly do not accept it, but the doctor only discovers this if he takes time to listen to his patient and to observe her reactions. Women who, for example, do not object to a hysterectomy may experience severe anxiety when faced with the possibility of a mastectomy. The uterus is not a visible organ. Many women do not even know what it looks like. But they know their breasts very well. They can see them and feel them; their breasts form an integral part of their body image.

Without going into a psychological interpretation of the function of the breast, which may be compared in some ways with that of the male sex organ, it must be pointed out that the removal of a breast always leads to a serious change in a woman's body image. She may lose the ability to express her femininity following a mastectomy and it is often hard to say

67

whether the major psychological problems resulting from mastectomy occur in the woman's relationship with herself or in the relationship with her partner.

Chardot (1968) studied the psychological consequences of the Halsted operation in 104 women, 95 of whom answered his questionnaire.

His data concerning prostheses are particularly interesting:

– only 18 women were not using prostheses. These were in particular those women whose other breast was small.
– 17 women had made for themselves a kind of 'stuffing' in their brassiere.
– 61 women used an external prosthesis.

Clearly most women want to appear as normal as possible and to hide their mutilation as much as possible. Of the 95 patients interviewed by Chardot, 47 stated that they accepted the removal of their breast as an inevitable evil. Of the other 48 women who underwent the operation, 21 regarded themselves irretrievably maimed.

The attitude of others, and of the partner in particular, is undoubtedly a factor of major importance, though of the remainder of the patients who had accepted the loss of their breast only 14 were aware of the favourable influence that their husbands had had on this.

It must therefore be said that therapists should do everything possible to avoid or to limit the psychological sequelae resulting from amputation of the breast for breast cancer.

Plastic surgery is only one of several therapeutic possibilities and it should never be the only one which is considered. Although it is believed that plastic surgery is harmless, this is not proven beyond doubt.

Another problem is the belief that, in case of carcinoma of the breast, reconstruction should not take place immediately following the mastectomy. In mutilating surgery on the face and/or the neck the approach is different because reconstruction takes place during the same operation at which malignant tissue is removed.

As far as the results are concerned, it is of course impossible to reach aesthetic perfection.

ON WHOM TO OPERATE?

Plastic surgery should be reserved for those patients whose chances of survival are good. Not all authors accept this point of view and some surgeons reconstruct breasts without taking the patient's chances of survival into account.

Breast reconstruction should only be considered beneficial for those patients whose life expectancy is comparable with that of healthy women of the same age. In those cases the procedure may be of great help.

On the basis of a detailed study of the 5 years' survival rates of 1046 patients who were treated in the Institute Gustave Roussy we can, with a certain degree of confidence, offer to perform breast reconstruction on patients who have the following types of tumours:

T1 tumours, if conservative therapy has not been effective	(T1 < 2 cm)
T2 tumours	(T2 = 2–5 cm)
T3 tumours	(T3 = 5–7 cm)

The presence or absence of metastases in the axillary nodes is very important. In patients with T1 type tumours where metastases had been found in these nodes, the 5-year survival rate decreased from 94% to 82%. In patients with T2 type nodes where metastases were found in their axillary nodes, the survival rate dropped from 87% to 67%.

WHEN TO OPERATE?

If it has been decided that reconstruction of the breast should be undertaken the next important question is how long after mastectomy this should be done. Some authors are in favour of early reconstruction. This, however, seems illogical and even dangerous. The period of time considered necessary before complete recovery is certain is 5 years. Survival rate curves, however, show that there is very little difference between the 3 years' survival rate and the 5-year survival rate.

It is therefore reasonable to wait until 3 years after the mastectomy is carried out, provided that the possibility of breast reconstruction at a later stage was discussed with the patient before her operation. The patient is thus given hope for the future. To be aware that a reconstruction procedure might be possible later gives the patient much support during the difficult period in which she has to learn to accept the loss of a breast. Even if the subsequent appearance of metastases excludes the feasibility of such a procedure, then the patient will still have received much consolation from the hope that it could be done at a later stage and it could even have helped her to accept the need for the loss of her breast.

To give a summary of the various therapeutic measures regarded as non-mutilating treatment is not necessary. It should only be pointed out that certain women, after they have been informed about the diagnosis and the need for an amputation, even if they are well aware of the dangers, still prefer to seek help from those therapists who treat breast cancer by non-surgical means alone, however far advanced it may be.

TECHNIQUE OF THE OPERATION

The aim of a breast reconstruction is to create a mass where the breast was situated and which resembles its appearance. It must be accepted however that it will not be possible to reconstruct a perfect breast. The areola and the nipple should also be reconstructed, although the latter is of less importance. Reconstruction of a breast always necessitates obtaining additional skin tissue. How this has to be done depends on the way in which the mastectomy was carried out. Can skin grafts be used for this purpose and if so, can this be done following a Halsted operation and after radiotherapy?

Two techniques are available, a skin flap can be obtained from the area adjacent to the operation site or skin can be grafted by means of a two-step procedure. In order to give the breast substance, the skin pouch which has been constructed needs to be filled. This can be done with a prosthesis, but a different material or a combination of the two can also be used.

If sufficient skin is available, it is usual to implant a prosthesis. This is not often possible, however, because in most cases much of the skin has been removed during the mastectomy. Shortage of skin, and in addition the application of post-operative radiotherapy, can make the technique of the operation very complicated.

The patient often objects to the use of a prosthesis and in that case a piece of omentum is used to fill the pouch which has been created by means of a skin graft.

Many different techniques are described in the literature because perfection has not yet been reached. It should be frankly acknowledged that the aesthetic results, whatever technique is used, are still far from perfect. The erogenous function of the breast, moreover, can never be restored.

But even though the function of the breast can never be restored, the recreation of the shape of the breast should always be attempted. This is what the patients want when they ask for a breast reconstruction. The surgeon himself is not always completely satisfied with his results from an aesthetic point of view, but most of the patients seem to be happy with them and this must always be the aim of the plastic surgeon.

Reference

Chardot, C. and Reilly, A. (1968). Séquelles acutelles et retentissement psychologique de l'opération de Halsted. *Presse Med.*, **76**, 1813

Discussion

Wenderlein: It is strange that, although with proper screening methods we can find very small tumours, surgeons still perform the Halsted operation even in those cases where this is not necessary.

Baruch: It will require much re-education to change this. I am afraid that we will be confronted with unnecessary Halsted operations until well into the next decade. Doctors, particularly male ones, have great difficulty in understanding the implications, both psychological and physical, of this operation to women.

Metze: In a hospital in Moscow where the whole surgical staff was female, mastectomies were considerably less radical.

Juret: Some surgeons use tissue of the vaginal wall to reconstruct a nipple. What is your opinion about this procedure?

Baruch: When I reconstruct a breast I have two objectives: I want to recreate the shape of the breast and I want to restore the function of the breast as far as this is possible. The nipple plays a role in sexual arousal, but only very few women ask the plastic surgeon to perform a nipple reconstruction as well. Either they do not want to undergo further surgery and regard the reconstruction of shape as satisfactory, or they presume rightly that a reconstructed nipple, whatever tissue would be used, will never be able to play the same role in sexual relationships as the real nipple did.

van Keep: Do you suggest that the plastic surgeon should operate on the breast rather than the general surgeon? Or should the plastic surgeon be present during the operation to indicate which tissues should be saved?

Baruch: Neither. The primary requirements at the moment of the mastectomy are dictated by the rules of oncology. I think, however, that the plastic surgeon should be involved in the discussion of the therapeutic strategy for a particular patient. We have adopted this approach in our hospital and the radiotherapist is also involved.

Metze: You said that your patients were satisfied with the results of the reconstruction. Do you have any data comparing, for example, sexual relationships after reconstruction compared with those where no reconstruction was done?

Baruch: No, my statement was based on purely clinical observation. We have now just started a more systematic approach.

Maguire: I know of some women whose husbands pressured them into having a reconstruction or an implant. Afterwards these husbands are usually not satisfied with the results and they may press their wives to have even further cosmetic surgery. Unrealistically, they want the breast to be exactly as it was before.

Baruch: I agree that the husband's pressure on his wife to ask for a reconstruction must be recognized. It is a complicating factor, particularly in long-standing relationships as found in cancer patients. The implant of a prosthesis is much easier, from the psychological point of view, in a young woman with hypoplasia of the breast. These women request the implantation of a prosthesis for their own reasons, often even before they have a partner. The future partner simply has to accept the result.

van den Heuvel: I still wonder why women should ask for a breast reconstruction. I can imagine that they would like a new breast but that is very different from what can be offered. How do you explain to these women the possible outcome of a reconstruction procedure?

Baruch: It is difficult to describe to a patient all the factors that may influence the result of her mastectomy. It is less difficult to inform women about the possible results of a reconstruction, because this is more predictable. Of course one must be honest and not create illusions, but in the end it is the patient who has to make up her mind and take the final decision.

9
Psychological Problems Related to the Conservative Treatment of Breast Cancer

P. JURET

During the last 10 years, conservative methods of treatment of breast cancer have gradually come to prevail. Most oncologists consider this change an important advance, since it enables some women to keep their breasts while it still provides effective treatment for their cancer. However, simplistic reasoning must be avoided with regard to limited surgical procedures. The related psychological aspects are the subject of this paper.

The original title suggested to me was: 'The reactions of women after breast surgery, especially after conservative treatment'.

I should like to broaden this subject to include the psychological problems faced by the oncologist and the surgeon.

Let us therefore consider:

1. The psychological problems of the oncologist and the surgeon;
2. The phychological problems of the patients.

THE PSYCHOLOGICAL PROBLEMS OF THE ONCOLOGIST AND OF THE SURGEON

During the first half of this century, Halsted's operation, with or without subsequent radiotherapy or removal of the ovaries, was regarded as the only acceptable method of treatment. '. . . Comme l'ont montré les premiers Halsted en Amérique et Banks en Angleterre, il faut opérer très largement . . .

73

La majorité des chirurgiens de tous les pays ont adopté actuellement la technique proposée par ces auteurs' (Lecène et Lenormant, 1928).*

. . . 'Le dogme fondamental est le rejet absolu de toute opération partielle; seule l'intervention très large doit être envisagée . . . Les bases théoriques de cette intervention large ont été posées par Halsted dès 1889 . . .' (Menegaux et Mathey, 1941).†

. . . 'Le cancer du sein de la femme au stade I relève de la chirurgie . . . amputation de Halsted plus ou moins modifiée mais comportant toujours un sacrifice cutané large, l'ablation des pectoraux, le curage complet de l'aisselle . . .' (Léger, 1953).‡

Over the years however, it became obvious that Halsted's operation did not represent the ideal solution as had been expected; despite increased experience of the surgeons, despite the introduction of radiotherapy into the arsenal of complementary means of treatment, despite campaigns urging women with lumps in their breasts to have themselves examined and treated without delay, a large number of patients, their breasts removed according to the classical doctrine, continued to die as a result of their cancer, sometimes from local recurrences, but more often from the effects of metastases.

Modifications of Halsted's original technique were then developed. Some surgeons tried to perfect it by looking for possible sites of neoplastic tissue in other than the axillary lymph nodes.

This led to the extension of the operation to two, three or four further areas, and removal, in addition to the axillary nodes, of the internal mammary, the supra-clavicular and even the superior mediastinal nodes . . . On the whole, these 'supra-radical' procedures did not achieve the hoped-for results. The disillusion which followed found expression in the report presented by Redon and Verhaeghe to the 70e Congrès Français de Chirurgie: '. . . On est d'ailleurs frappé, à dépouiller les statistiques, par une sorte de seuil autour de 60 pour cent qui répond à la survie à 5 ans des séries comprenant le "tout-venant" . . .'§

A new school of thought then appeared whose aim was to obtain this threshold of 60% 5-year survival with less mutilating operations than Halsted's procedure such as mastectomies without removal of pectoralis major and mastectomies without axillary node removal and various types of

---

* 'As first demonstrated by Halsted in America and Banks in England, a very extensive operation is necessary. The great majority of surgeons, all over the world, have now adopted the technique suggested by the authors.'
† 'The fundamental dogma is total rejection of all partial operations; only very few extensive procedures should be considered suitable . . . and their basic features have been enunciated by Halsted as early as 1889.'
‡ Carcinoma of the female breast (stage I) is to be treated surgically . . . Halsted's amputation, modified to a greater or a lesser extent, but always involving removal of large areas of skin, removal of the pectoral muscles, and complete curettage of the axilla . . .'
§ 70th Convention of the French Surgical Association: 'Statistics show the existence of a kind of threshold around 60%. It corresponds to the 5-year survival rate of groups which include all patients.'

tumour removal. The most extreme attitude is that of La Fondation Curie (Paris), which tries to treat breast cancer with irradiation only, reserving subsequent surgery for those cases in which radiation has failed to cure the patient.

Over the last 20 years, this less mutilating form of treatment has gradually come to the fore, but some surgeons still consider it 'scandalous' not to give patients the benefit of Halsted's operation which they regard as a gospel that allows no heretical interpretations. A proponent of this point of view is Haagensen who, in 1973, entitled an editorial on these conservative methods: 'A great leap backward in the treatment of carcinoma of the breast'.

It has become impossible to ignore the plight of oncologists who are torn between the doctrine of Halsted and his followers on the one hand and current conservative tendencies on the other. Even now, I know surgeons who feel extremely uncomfortable when faced with breast cancer: they knew very well how to treat it 20 years ago but they no longer know how to treat it at present.

THE PSYCHOLOGICAL PROBLEMS OF THE PATIENT

The psychological problems of the patient must of course be foremost in our consideration. It is beyond question that to be allowed to keep her breast when it is affected by cancer represents a significant advantage for a woman, particularly if she is young. I shall not enlarge on this as it is a matter of common sense. Nevertheless, the essentials of the problem must be carefully weighed, in order not to give a woman false hopes which will be contradicted by the facts.

It must not be forgotten that conservative treatment necessitates an extremely rigorous follow-up for many years and does not eliminate the possibility that a mastectomy may have to be performed later if the tumour resumes its local growth. Furthermore, many tumours, for reasons to be discussed later, are not suitable for conservative surgery.

The following principles must be emphasized:

I. Conservative surgery should be done only when it makes sense from the aesthetic point of view. To try to conserve part of the breast, even if two-thirds of it would have to be removed during the course of tumourectomy, would be absurd. Such a procedure would leave the patient with a mammary monstrosity which is worse than a mastectomy scar. From the patients I have followed up I took some pictures showing both, tumour removal with acceptable results (Figures 9.1 and 9.2) and deformations of the breast, such as strabismus of the nipple (Figures 9.3 and 9.4).

At a recent symposium organized by 'la Fondation Curie' in Paris, most of the speakers agreed that conservative treatment should in general only be applied to tumours smaller than 3 cm. Interpretation of this figure must

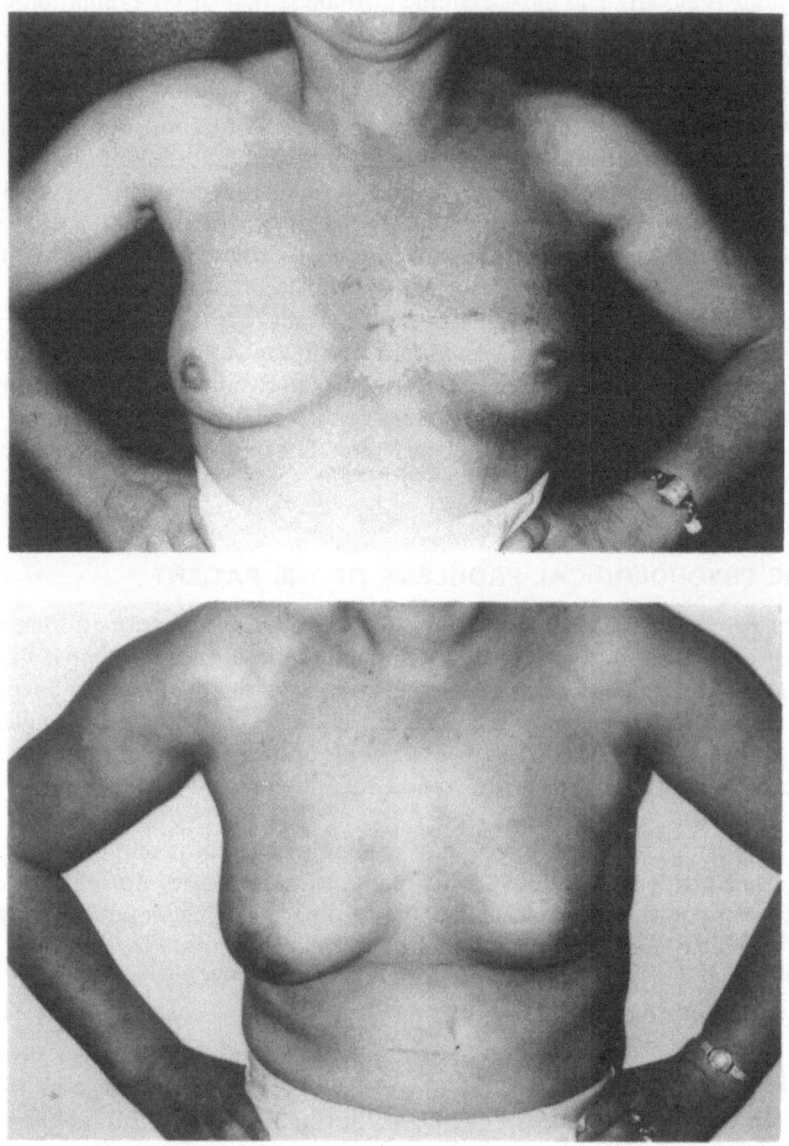

Figures 9.1 and 9.2 Tumourectomies for breast cancer – acceptable results

of course be flexible. If a breast is large, a tumour of 4 cm could be acceptably treated by local removal only while, on the other hand, removal of a tumour of 3 cm would be unacceptable if the woman had very small breasts.

It should also be mentioned that breasts which have been treated with

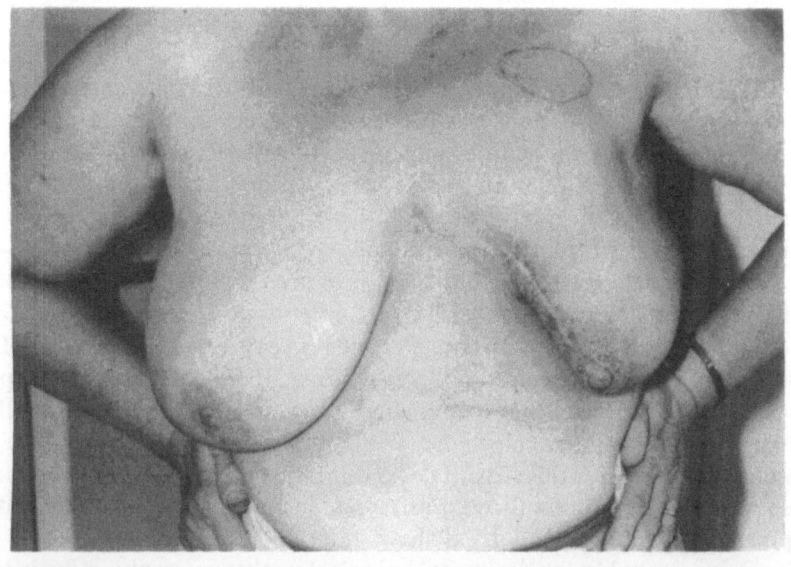
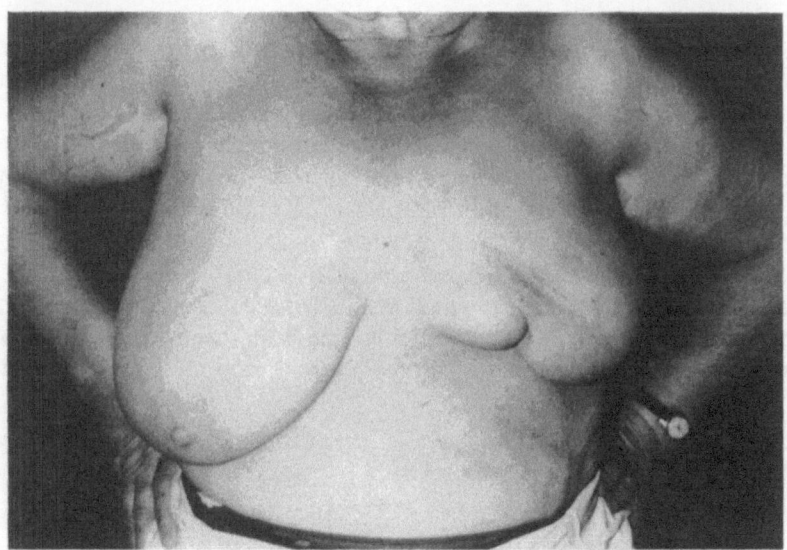

Figures 9.3 and 9.4 Tumourectomies for breast cancer – questionable results

local tumour removal involving much loss of tissue can no longer be fitted with a brassiere. The reason is that the breast tissue which has been left behind prevents a prosthesis from being used to give the brassiere its normal outline.

77

II. The woman who wants to be treated conservatively must be unequivocally informed of the need for a close follow-up for a long period of time during which frequent mammographies will have to be done. She should also be told of the possibility that mastectomy may still become necessary if it becomes apparent that conservative treatment has failed. All published series of conservative procedures include cases where a subsequent mastectomy was required, so it would be dishonest to hide this possibility from the patient. This consideration must weigh heavily when the anxiety, induced by different forms of treatment is evaluated. Although I do not dispute the shattering effect that a mastectomy can have on a woman, I can also testify to the fact that many women who have undergone a local tumourectomy are subjected to a real and prolonged ordeal because of their constant fear that the tumour has not been completely removed. I remember several women who told me bluntly that they would have preferred losing their breast if they had known that keeping their breast would imply such a long follow-up and so much suspense. For this reason I also think that the oncologist should not insist on a conservative procedure if a patient is clearly not interested in keeping her breast, particularly if she is elderly.

These are probably the main psychological problems resulting from conservative surgery in the treatment of breast cancer. I am convinced that conservative procedures represent a step forward, provided that certain conditions are met. It must be carefully considered whether conservative treatment will suit the individual patient. These methods must not be thought of as universal remedies which are applicable to all forms of breast cancer and to each patient. The patient must be warned of the imperative need for follow-up if her breast is preserved and of the possibility that mastectomy may still be required later.

Finally, the patient must be psychologically capable of coping with the agony of suspense. The ordeal which results from conservative treatment is, in my opinion, for some women harder to bear than the distress which would have been caused by a total mastectomy performed as a primary procedure.

References

Haagensen, C. D. (1973). A great leap backward in the treatment of carcinoma of the breast. *J. Am. Med. Assoc.*, **224**, 1181
Lecène, P. and Lenormant, C. (1928). Maladies chirurgicales de la glande mammaire. In: *Précis de Pathologie Chirurgicale*, 5th ed. (Paris)
Léger, L. (1953). Tumeurs malignes du sein. In: *Prat. Med. Chir.*, 4th ed. (Paris)
Menegaux, G. and Mathey, J. (1941). Néoplasmes mammaires et perimammaires. In: *Encyclop. Med. Chir.: Gynécologie et mamelle* (Paris)
Redon, H. and Verhaeghe, M. (1968). Indications therapeutiques dans le cancer du sein. Paper presented at the *70th Convention of the French Surgical Association* (Paris)

Discussion

Wenderlein: You have not dealt with other forms of therapy, such as chemotherapy and hormone therapy. Yet these should also be considered.

Juret: Of course one should keep all possible forms of therapy in mind. I do not think that post-operative chemotherapy is of much benefit to patients who are over 50 years old. Chemotherapy is also quite an ordeal for the patient; it involves much stress, both physically and psychologically. In fact, chemotherapy is at present mainly reserved for those patients in whom much axillary involvement is found and for whom the prognosis is poor. Most oncologists are nowadays also rather sceptical about the value of 'prophylactic castration'.

Wenderlein: I believe that hormone therapy has a definite place in the treatment of elderly women. Progestogens can be very useful in the management of old ladies for whom the quality of life is perhaps more important than 5-year survival rates.

Juret: Each patient requires an individual decision. Some women would rather have a mastectomy then be forced to become a 'satellite' of an oncological unit. In some patients one reaches the conclusion – after weighing all aspects of the situation – that a tumourectomy is indicated. In other cases, for example patients with a low level of intelligence, a total mastectomy could well be the most satisfactory method of treatment, as these patients are often unlikely to attend the frequent follow-up procedures which are needed after more conservative forms of treatment.

Baruch: Many of the surgeons who do tumourectomies also have a psychological problem. After the operation, feelings of doubt develop. They become uncertain whether all malignant tissue has in fact been removed. They therefore decide that the patient should also have radiotherapy and, believe me, the result of cobalt radiation following tumourectomy is not a pleasant sight. I much prefer a complete mastectomy to this form of treatment.

Juret: I agree with you. As I mentioned in my paper, there is ample evidence that a complete mastectomy is in some cases a more satisfactory method of treatment than simple tumourectomy followed by radiotherapy. Factors which must be taken into account before it is decided which procedure to follow include the size of the tumour and the age and personality of the patient.

van Keep: Although many forms of conservative treatment may be an improvement, I think that for the time being, and until their real value is established, they should only be used by those who are experienced in their use.

Maguire: A study at Guy's Hospital in London revealed that there was a greater risk of local recurrence if conservative treatment was used. Such a recurrence is very alarming to the patient. If the affected breast is not removed, there may be women who are worried that some of the tumour has been left behind.

10
Psychological Reactions of Breast Cancer Patients to Radiotherapy

KARIN GYLLENSKÖLD

BACKGROUND

From 1971 to 1973 a group of women with breast cancer was studied by the author from the psychological point of view at Radiumhemmet, Karolinska Sjukhuset, Stockholm. In 1971 a medical study had been carried out at Radiumhemmet involving a great number of breast cancer patients.

The 21 patients interviewed in this study were recruited, in a randomized way, from this larger population. To be included in the medical study, patients had to meet eight criteria:

1. The patient had to be a woman.
2. The patient had to have cytologically verified carcinoma of the breast.
3. There had to be a possibility of treatment by a modified radical mastectomy.
4. The local extension of the tumour had to fall within stages I and II according to the TNM system of classification. Patients with infected tumours were excluded.
5. The patient had to be less than 70 years old.
6. The patient should not have malignancy in both breasts.
7. The patient should not be pregnant or have had a delivery or an abortion within the preceding six months.
8. The tumour should not have been treated previously.

OBJECTIVES

The purpose of our study has been to improve understanding of the psychological processes peculiar to women who receive treatment for cancer of the breast. Apart from the psychological aspects of radiation treatment the study involved research into the psychological and sexual meaning of the female breast, breast development and breast feeding. Delay in terms of psychological defence mechanisms, the psychological implications resulting from confirmation of the diagnosis of mammary carcinoma and from mastectomy were studied, as well as the phenomenon of phantom breast in terms of body image, body ego and of bereavement. Finally the psychological reactions to cancer, 'the illness that is more dreaded by man than any other', were analysed and described (Gyllensköld, 1976). This paper will deal with the psychological aspects of radiation therapy only.

METHOD

Patients in the study were interviewed as follows:

– immediately after they had been told that they had cancer of the breast;
– 1 week after they had been told that they had cancer of the breast;
– 3 weeks after mastectomy;
– at the end of their radiation treatment;
– 6 months after they had been given the diagnosis;
– 12 months after they had been given the diagnosis;
– 24 months after they had been given the diagnosis.

Interviews usually lasted 1 hour and were tape recorded with the patient's permission. The total contents of the tapes were then typed out. The interview was carried out in the form of 'free talks' and after some time patients felt free to introduce any topic they wanted to discuss.

Table 10.1   Patients who had radiotherapy

	Group A patients Pre-op	Group B patients Post-op
Number	6	6
Age	M = 56(±7)	M = 53(±7)
Marital status		
Married	2	5
Unmarried	1	—
Divorced	2	1
Widow	1	—
Children		
Yes	5	6
No	1	—
Occupational work		
Yes	4	3
No	2	3
Education		
Primary school	2	2
High school	4	4

PATIENTS IN THE STUDY

Of the 21 women in the study six had radiation treatment before (group A) and six after (group B) their modified radical mastectomy. There were some small, negligible differences between patients in group A and group B concerning background variables such as age and marital status, as shown in Table 10.1.

RESULTS

Other studies on the psychological experiences of patients undergoing radiotherapy are scarce or non-existent. Since this study only concerns a total of 12 patients, great caution has been taken with the analysis of the data and the results which are presented here are therefore of a descriptive nature.

Questions about radiation treatment

All patients asked questions on radiation treatment before they were due to receive it. The questions asked mostly had a matter-of-fact quality, such as:

– Does it hurt?
– Will it leave scars or other marks?
– How long does it take?
  (a) the whole period of treatment?
  (b) each single application?
– Will I be able to work while I receive treatment?
– How will the treatment influence my whole body?
– Will I become depressed or in other ways psychologically affected by the treatment?
– Will I be sterile after the treatment?
– Will the radiation remain within my body and for how long?
– Will I be dangerous to other people during the treatment?
– Will I be able to sunbathe after the treatment?
– How will the treatment be administered to me?

Patients are usually not well informed before they receive different types of medical treatment (Egbert et al., 1964; Bard et al., 1955).

After the results of this study were published, Radiumhemmet has provided an information folder for patients who need treatment. In this folder questions like the ones mentioned above are discussed and answered.

Three of the 12 patients interviewed continued to work – either full- or part-time – during the whole of their period of treatment. Two of these patients received post-operative and one received pre-operative treatment. Two of these patients had had some difficulties with their doctors, who did not approve of their remaining at work during treatment.

Patients' fears of radiation treatment

Before their treatment, all 12 patients were afraid of radiotherapy. However, they tried not to show this to the hospital staff because they thought that doctors, nurses, and radiotherapy assistants:

– expected patients not to be afraid;
– did not like frightened patients;
– would interpret patients' fears in terms of mistrust of their competence to handle the radiotherapy equipment properly;
– would interpret patients' fears in terms of 'weakness', 'worthlessness', or 'immaturity'.

Most of the patients had known or heard of other women who had received radiotherapy. These women had talked about it in terms such as 'being burnt altogether', 'becoming a nervous wreck', 'unable to breathe'. This, of course, had made them even more frightened. But the reason that they were frightened was also related to their various preconceived ideas – either true or false – about radiation treatment.

Patients' concepts of radiation treatment

Patients believed that radiation treatment could be dangerous in different ways. It could be harmful to the skin as well as to the heart and the lungs. It might even cause the growth of more cancer. One patient said that she had started taking off her watch at night, which she had never done before. She laughed about it but said: 'Even though I know that I am being stupid, I do believe that having had those radiating figures close to the skin for more than 40 years cannot have been very healthy. Oh, I don't think they caused my cancer, but still . . .'

Another woman said: 'High voltage station* – it sounds like the electric chair. It may be a convenient word to use for the technicians, but to me . . . high voltage . . . I immediately thought of those signs "Danger. High tension. Do not touch". Since I was a child I was taught not to go close to those things because you might get killed. If you receive such a current, you are finished, dead!'

Some patients related 'irradiation' with 'atom bombs' or with 'very strong explosions'. One woman said: 'I thought: radium, that kills – if it is not under control. Dangerous. There was a moment of . . . radium can murd . . . kill you.'

A few patients thought that radiation might be harmful to their genes: 'I don't know how far medicine has advanced, but if a doctor would tell me that radiation treatment is not dangerous for "the next generation" then I would not believe him.'

---

* The name of the radiotherapy department at Radiumhemmet.

Some patients believed that radiation treatment influenced their psyche: 'Well, I couldn't think . . . thoughts just stopped inside my head. I tried to count, one, two, three . . . but then it was impossible for me to continue. I thought it had to do with the treatment, but perhaps it was only my nerves . . .' Another woman said: 'It is strange, but it is in the head too, and in the whole of my body. I cannot concentrate at all.' And another: 'It makes you feel cowardly and tired. I don't believe that it is the rays, but still there must be something that affects the psyche.'

One patient believed that the treatment had given her a greater resistance to infectious diseases.

Finally, a few patients were afraid that the radiation would stay within their bodies and that they might pass it on to other people: 'What about my family . . . shall I be dangerous to them?' – 'I hope I am not a danger to others, but I have had this funny feeling, a sort of prickling . . . Well, it could not possibly be strong enough to hurt somebody else . . .'

Experiences while lying underneath the apparatus in the treatment room

Most patients reported that at one time or another they had experienced feelings of panic while they were having treatment. This could have been expected after learning about their fears beforehand and about their concepts of radiation treatment. Patients tried to cope with their feelings of panic in different ways and none of them had to have their treatment interrupted because of panic, although this did happen a few times with other patients at Radiumhemmet.

'Oh, it was like torture, I felt panic . . . I wanted to scream, get up and run away,' or 'I became very panicky, but then I talked slowly to myself to calm down.'

Alone in the treatment room, confronted with the huge machines, many patients also experienced strong feelings of helplessness and of being dependent. They were, for instance, afraid that the staff might forget to turn the machines off. All patients knew that the staff could watch them through closed-circuit television from the control room, but they would have liked to have had their own audio-communication with the staff as well.

Many patients were afraid that the radiotherapists would suddenly lose control of the equipment in one way or another, so that the machines would give too high a dose, explode, break down, or even fall upon them. 'I have the feeling that it might fall on me. It must weigh tons, and if . . . well, it would flatten you like a pancake. And after that you wouldn't exist any more' (laughs). 'It is big, isn't it?'

One doctor had once said to a patient that the radiotherapy equipment behaved like a 'primadonna'. When she was later asked about her reaction to that she replied: 'Well, I thought it would do things the way it wished to.

Suddenly it would start irradiating at a terrible speed instead of remaining calm. You know what a primadonna is like . . . extreme things can happen . . .'

Another patient said: 'I often saw a man who looked like an engineer . . . I had to wait almost every day . . . there was always something wrong with the machines. The staff talked about control, but I thought that if those machines break down so easily that a man has to repair them every day . . . they must be very unreliable . . .'

Patients were afraid that members of staff might administer too high a dose because of mistakes in their calculations: 'They really have responsible jobs, those who sit there counting dosages. They could make a mistake. That is human, it happens everywhere.' 'You often find evidence that the human factor causes catastrophes and disasters. One is not safe anywhere.'

In spite of all negative feelings referred to above, patients also felt the positive experience of having been taken care of and of receiving professional help for their malignant disease. The patients' longing to get better and their faith in medicine, together with the support they received from the members of staff and from their own coping or defence mechanisms, had made things easier for them during their treatment. One patient said during the interview:

'I was very frightened and felt unsafe.'

'How did you cope with those feelings?'

'I swallowed . . .' (laughs).

'You swallowed?'

'Yes, oh yes. You learn to do that as a child. But . . . I went for further treatment every time because I wanted to get better. Doctors say that radiation treatment helps and obviously it does.'

Examples of psychological coping mechanisms used by patients while receiving radiotherapy

Patients used different coping strategies to try to escape from feelings of anxiety while they received treatment. Suppression was most frequently used. For instance, patients mentally recited nursery rhymes and counted or recited poetry or hymns to themselves.

One woman made use of reaction formation and said: 'Oh, it made me feel full of energy . . . gave me the feeling of getting fresh air. That's the way I felt.'

Another said: 'We joked a lot, one does when it is . . . well, I do, anyway . . . I joked and said "Now I am getting a nice sun tan" . . .' (laughs).

'But as a matter of fact . . .?'

'One doesn't like it . . . I really didn't.'

Denial was another coping device used. The woman who in her interview had compared irradiation with the electric chair said later in that same interview: 'Actually, it was not distressing at all . . . I didn't feel a bit worried.' Another woman said: 'I really didn't feel I was going to a hospital' (for her daily treatment). 'I just sort of dropped in before work.'

A few patients used repression some time after they had finished their radiotherapy: 'It passed so quickly. It is almost as if I never went there . . . I have . . . erased it in some way . . .'

Comparisons between patients who had had radiotherapy before and patients who had radiotherapy after their mastectomy

Patients who received radiation treatment before their operation probably had a more difficult time psychologically than patients who had it post-operatively. One reason was that they still had to undergo an operation after they had finished with their radiotherapy.

Some found this very disturbing and were afraid that the cancer could have spread further because their breast had not immediately been removed. But at the same time, these patients believed that those women who had had their operations first were worse off than they themselves were, because the others had had tumours which were so dangerous that they had to be removed at once.

On the other hand, patients who had received post-operative radiotherapy thought that those women who were irradiated before their operation were worse off, since the tumours of these women would otherwise have become inoperable. Patients who did not receive any radiotherapy believed this to be a sign that their tumours were less dangerous than those of the patients who had needed radiotherapy.

These phenomena can be regarded as a manifestation of the need these women had to interpret their own situation as favourably as possible whatever the form of treatment was they received.

The following table gives a schematic assessment of how patients 'felt' during the whole period of radiotherapy:

Table 10.2   Patient's feelings during radiotherapy

	Pre-operative radiotherapy	Post-operative radiotherapy	Total number of patients
Worried, afraid, feelings of anxiety	6	6	12
Very tired	6	4	10
Apathetic	2	1	3
Unmotivated bouts of crying	2	—	2
Dizziness	2	—	2
Hyperactivity	—	1	1

CONCLUSIONS

The number of patients that took part in this study is small. Yet the findings seem to have some general validity as they have been recognized by staff members of different radiology departments of hospitals throughout Sweden.

Those who work in these departments at times seem to be unaware of the profound fears of their patients. This is due to two sets of circumstances. One is that patients seem unwilling to reveal their true feelings and fantasies to the members of staff. The other is that members of the staff themselves use coping mechanisms, such as suppression, denial and reaction-formation, to manage their own anxiety as well as that of their patients.

Radiotherapy is not only physically but also psychologically stressing. To make radiotherapy easier for them, the patients should be given more and preferably written, information about this form of treatment and they should be given the opportunity to psychologically work through the different emotions and notions which are related to this form of treatment.

One of the most important conclusions is that the members of staff of radiotherapy units should receive adequate training in psychology and that proper supervision should be provided (Cousland, 1973).

References

Bard, M. and Sutherland, A. M. (1955). Psychological impact of cancer and its treatment. *Cancer*, **8** (4), 656

Cousland, H. C. (1973). Some thoughts on the training of radiographers. *Radiography, May*, **39**, 136

Egbert, D. L., Battit, E. G., Welch, E. C. and Bartlett, K. M. (1964). Reduction of postoperative pain by encouragement and instruction of patients. *N. Engl. J. Med.*, **270**, 825

Gyllensköld, K. (1976). *Visst blir man rädd . . . Samtal med kvinnor som behandlats för bröstcancer*. (Stockholm: Forum)

Discussion

van Brederode: Would the best time to give a woman information about radiation therapy be when she is told that she may need a mastectomy?

Gyllensköld: I think that she should receive this information when it is likely that she will need radiotherapy, but I think that it should be given again later because she will probably have forgotten the details. Before the actual start of therapy she should receive further information, this time with all the data which apply to her own particular case.

Metze: Cancer, for most patients, is a mysterious disease. It is something beyond their control, something that grows within them. I wonder how much radiotherapy adds to this feeling.

Gyllensköld: The equipment certainly gives the patients an impression of magic. The staff members who operate this equipment are looked upon as 'omnipotent', almost as representatives of God, who have been given powers to decide on life and death. We noticed that the staff of radiotherapy departments receive presents from their patients much more often than staff members of other hospital departments. It is as if their patients are trying to please them: 'Please help me so that those machines will not do anything they should not while I am there.'

Vermost: Should we not go even further and inform the whole population about the basic principles of radiotherapy?

Gyllensköld: The patient's relatives should in any case receive this information and I agree that it would be a very good thing if the whole population could be informed through the mass media.

Humphrey: I became aware, while listening to this paper, that notices in a hospital may be frightening indeed to patients. We are perhaps too much involved in trying to help the individual patient to be able to see the problems of 'patients' as a group. Would there be any advantage in having group discussions with members of the staff to draw attention to such problems?

Gyllensköld: I had some informal discussions about this. Members of staff use all kinds of defence mechanisms and deny that many of these problems exist. I think that they find it also difficult to handle their own emotional problems.

Maguire: Sometimes senior members of staff do not like their juniors to see that they also have emotional problems. They may, therefore, resist the idea of staff meetings. But I agree that staff meetings are beneficial.

Gyllensköld: Radiotherapy constitutes a very upsetting form of treatment for the patient. She has to overcome an enormous psychological stress and she feels very tired, at times exhausted. To be lying underneath such big radiotherapy equipment is very threatening. It all seems so mysterious and magical.

C.M.: My own experiences were like that. When I went for treatment the first time the day had changed into night and I felt completely abandoned. I had to cope with all my problems alone. Treatment lasted two months and I felt exhausted. For the first time ever I needed to go to sleep after lunch.

Maguire: Part of the fatigue is of course due to the effect of radiation itself, but the psychological stress must use up much energy too.

Gyllensköld: To come back to the members of the staff, they cannot and also should not try to remove every problem for the patient. Before the operation, for example, the patient should have a certain amount of fear. The staff should allow their patients to be frightened and to express this. They should not tell their patients 'Don't be afraid, we will take care of everything', but they should say 'Tell us what you are afraid of, so that we can help you.'

Wenderlein: The patient could be supported in her loneliness by the use of two-way monitors, microphones and loudspeakers.

Gyllensköld: Well, this kind of equipment does exist, but the staff members switch it off because they do not want to be overheard by the patients when they discuss their own affairs.

11
Factors Affecting Participation in Cancer Screening Programmes

L. VERMOST

THE CASE FOR SCREENING PROGRAMMES

In Belgium early detection of cancer has, during the last 10 years and within the frameworks of anti-cancer programmes and preventive health care, developed into a very important area of public health. In spite of this relatively recent development, the 1966 budget of the Belgian Ministry of Public Health shows that the six University-based 'Early Cancer Detection Centres' in Belgium spent between them 32 million Belgian Francs ($800 000). This amount increased to 45 million Belgian Francs ($1 100 000) in 1971 and then fell back slightly to 30 million Belgian Francs ($750 000) in 1973. These centres are also expected to obtain additional funds from other sources, so that estimates of the yearly costs of cancer prevention are as high as 85 million Belgian Francs ($2 800 000). These centres organize and carry out mass-screening programmes, mostly in places of employment and in population centres. The majority of these 'Early Detection Centres' concentrates on screening programmes for cancer of the breast and cancer of the cervix. It has been estimated that about 100 000 individual screening procedures were carried out in 1972.

Participation in these mass-screening programmes varies, on average, from 20% to 40%, with a few extremes in either direction. Participation within homogeneous groups, such as industrial companies, is often as high as 60%.

The rate of detection of malignancy is constant at six per 1000. This means that 600 cases of early or advanced cancer were detected by means of these programmes in 1972.

Low participation figures constitute a problem both from the purely medical and from the socio-medical points of view. The solution to this problem, however, can only be found by workers in the field of behavioural sciences since additional insights into the problem can only be obtained from the study of the points of view of the populations concerned.

In other words, the correlation of the principles underlying the screening campaigns with the needs and attitudes of the 'consumers' should be examined. Therefore, the 'client-orientation' of this field of health care should be studied. This should explain the type of approach of this study used by the *Sociologisch Onderzoeksinstituut** (Sociological Research Institute).

FACTORS AFFECTING PARTICIPATION

Our *basic hypothesis* was that there are profound differences between the rationale from which these screening programmes were developed and the rationale of the target population (women from 30 to 65 years). Participation in preventive cancer screening might then be explained by the tendency of the participants to conform to the central values of the health services, for example, through education, or to adjust themselves to these central values as a result of social networks and information campaigns. Non-participation could then possibly be explained by basic differences between the values of the health services and those of the non-participants.

Our *study* focused on the comparison between participants and non-participants to test the above hypothesis. Its confirmation would imply that cancer screening facilities are used only by those people who can adjust their own values to those of the Health Services, which are derived from the specific rationale of this service.

Comparison of the participant and non-participant groups focused on two main sets of factors:

1. Behaviour and attitudes related to illness and health, termed the *health perspective*, which may either conform to or deviate from the basic philosophy of the screening programme.

2. *Socio-cultural data* such as age, education, social class and family status, which might explain a possible bridging of the cultural gap.

Central themes of the study were situational characteristics of age and social class (including education). There was clearly an inverse correlation between age and participation. Notably above the age of 55, participation fell sharply, while it was also relatively low in the lowest and the highest

---

* Part of the Catholic University of Leuven, where a research project on Socio-cultural Determinants of Health and Illness Behaviour was made possible by a grant from the FGWO, Brussels.

social classes. Participation in the screening programme was highest in the middle classes.

An important finding was that both age and social class factors were closely linked with indicators (situational characteristics as well as health perspective dimensions) of the concepts of social integration and activism. Young women and middle-class women were found to be better integrated socially and also to possess a more active attitude towards the control of illness and health, and this resulted in higher participation.

Thus both concepts, integration and activism, play an intermediate role between hard social data and health behaviour.

The *typical participant* in preventive cancer screening can be described as the young married woman with two or more children who has reached a certain level of education, who is socially well integrated and possesses a rational attitude towards illness and health, who is active in the field of health (and also has sufficient medical knowledge), who is capable of organizing and controlling her life, and who makes use of all facilities provided by modern science.

The *typical non-participant* can be described as the somewhat older woman with a small or maturing family, who has had little education, who has been more or less 'shelved' by society, who experiences illness with less rationality and less knowledge and who has a rather fatalistic attitude towards the events of life and an indifferent attitude towards remedies offered by medicine.

These findings seem to confirm the sometimes disputed 'middle-class theory', which suggests that middle-class behaviour represents a standard to live up to. In terms of cancer prevention, this would imply that participation in a mass-screening programme is desirable middle-class behaviour.

The middle-class model agrees very well with certain central values in mass-screening programmes. Several authors attribute three values to the 'medical institution', which are also of central importance to Western society.

These values, which can be recognized in any health service and therefore also in preventive cancer screening programmes for women, are: materialism, activism and instrumentalism.

Materialism

'Health and illness are reduced to objective categories, to be dealt with in rational terms.' In practice, this means that cancer is reduced to its objective, physically observable dimension and is stripped of any taboo, personal element or emotion. Because of this reduction the consumer is required to respond in equally rational terms.

The comparison of participants and non-participants shows a slight over-representation of non-rational *illness concepts* (religious, nature-orientated) among the non-participants.

This means that more people with concepts of illness that differ from the (rational) one incorporated in the preventive cancer screening programmes are found amongst non-participants than amongst participants. In the field of rational *medical knowledge*, the same tendency becomes apparent – there is less knowledge and, therefore, less familiarity with health care among non-participants.

Activism

'Medicine has succeeded in defeating poliomyelitis, measles and all kinds of epidemic diseases: therefore, cancer and other modern illnesses will soon be treated with equal success.' The same belief in total control of the environment, of illness and health, and of life in general, is also expected of the consumer. A comparison between participants and non-participants concerning their active or resigned attitude towards the problems of life in general and those of health in particular was made on the basis of the scales of Dean, which attempt to index feelings of *powerlessness* and *hopelessness*.

The two groups in the study showed clear differences, the non-participants registering the highest scores on both scales, which shows that they have in general a more fatalistic attitude towards life.

Preventive mass-screening thus seems to find a larger response amongst those groups of the population that tend to possess the activist attitude demanded by modern medicine.

Instrumentalism

'Medicine is able to provide the means which solve many of the problems of health and living, such as staying awake or being able to sleep and stimulating the appetite or reducing it. These remedies or instruments in our society are increasing in diversity and number, even to the point that many people tend to feel guilty when, for example, they have not taken preventive 'flu' injections. This instrumentalism, or shifting of attention from goal to means, may also be enforced (obligatory vaccinations, all kinds of tests).

Therefore, individuals or groups who have this instrumental attitude towards health and illness can be expected to participate more. Thus far, research data on these subjects are still lacking.

This is how the first results of our investigation have led to an evaluation of preventive cancer screening for women by means of mass-screening methods. The hypothesis that such mass-screening procedures, by incorporating some central values, evoke more responses from a certain type of consumer who conforms better to their underlying cultural pattern, seems to be provisionally confirmed. It is therefore safe to conclude that certain values and principles seem to be incorporated in preventive cancer screening, which determine in advance the size and nature of the clientele or participating group.

RECOMMENDATIONS

Two possibilities exist for the future: attempts may be made to increase participation by offering information to more people (for example, by better propaganda – and information – campaigns), or else the health facilities offered (in this case mass-screening) may be organized along different lines so as to take the differing rationales held by the population into account.

These two objectives do not entirely exclude each other, and it would be a mistake, at this stage of cancer prevention, to exclude either possibility. Nevertheless, we should be aware that mass-screening is only a means and not a goal in itself. In conceiving such campaigns, we should take into account that there are also other means to achieve the same end. Although, in the present phase of .cancer prevention, mass-screening plays the important roles of detection and of sensitization, we should ask ourselves whether many women (as well as men) would not be better off consulting their own doctor, so that mass-screening methods could be reserved for certain hard-to-reach risk groups.

Our first recommendation, therefore, is to give cancer detection and prevention a 'normal' place within the individuals' health and illness behaviour. The best means to obtain this are self-care and a personal doctor–patient relationship. Within this framework, the taboo surrounding cancer would be wiped out, and at the same time the illness would be 'dematerialized'.

Secondly, cancer detection should become incorporated within the structure of health education and should aim to obtain greater self-responsibility and increased activism. Perhaps emphasis should be shifted from the possibilities of medical achievement towards those of individual human achievement, and towards finding a better way to protect and sustain our own health through individual action (prevention, detection).

Finally, wherever mass-orientated campaigns remain useful, much attention should be given to information and motivation of the risk groups involved. To this end, it is best to use channels already present in the local community, such as associations and community development schemes. Posters and pamphlets will probably not suffice. Local health workers should be involved, directing their attention to individuals as well as to the group. The latter will probably be best reached through information meetings, although we should not expect too much from this approach.

CONCLUSION

This study showed that cancer detection programmes are capable of reaching only that part of the population whose life style conforms to the values of the campaign. Therefore, the main objective of cancer prevention and cancer detection programmes should be to become an integral part of the individual's own health and illness behaviour.

Discussion

Wenderlein: Our own data suggest that those women who remember when their breasts started to grow are also the ones who tend to perform regular self-examinations. This would suggest that self-examination should be taught at a very early stage.

Vermost: I agree entirely. Not only should the body be demystified, but also what may happen to it.

Juret: Our experience with screening programmes has been rather unfavourable. In one group of 990 women who were screened, no malignancy was found. These programmes are expensive in relation to their results. It remains of course very important to investigate women who have noticed something wrong with their breasts. As far as the high-risk groups are concerned, we should not underestimate the anxiety that our insistence on regular screening produces.

If a woman, whose mother had died from breast cancer, attends for screening and nothing is found, then this does not mean that nothing will be found the following year either.

Vermost: Doubts about the efficacy of large-scale screening methods are often expressed in various countries, but little is being done to replace them by better ones. Education of the population and of the medical profession is needed.

Wenderlein: When a patient at risk visits me for her annual check-up and I can tell her that nothing wrong has been found, I feel that I have reduced her anxiety, not increased it.

Vermost: The isolation of mass-screening from personal behaviour and education concerning health and illness creates either undue anxiety or false feelings of security.

Maguire: There is a psychological aspect to screening that is often overlooked. The woman who comes for screening expects to be rewarded for what she regards as good behaviour. She expects to be reassured that she is well but in some cases, when a tumour is found, the opposite happens.

A second point is that the success of screening programmes is tremendously enhanced if women can be approached personally.

Vermost: Another result of this person-to-person contact is that a socialization process is provoked. Even those women who are difficult to involve in any programme are encouraged to accept the values of the health services and of society.

12
Participants and Non-participants in a Mammography Mass-screening: Who is Who

W. J. A. VAN DEN HEUVEL

INTRODUCTION

Effectiveness of mass-screening for cancer depends on five factors at least: (1) incidence and history of the disease, (2) diagnostic sensitivity to avoid a significant number of false negatives and false positives, (3) therapies resulting in high long-term survival rates, (4) information and health education to motivate the largest possible number of people to participate, and (5) costs as a result of the four factors mentioned above in terms of money spent per person, organization needed, manpower, etc.

Studies concerning attitudes and information towards cancer have clearly shown how negative the image of cancer really is (van den Heuvel, 1977a). The word cancer provokes feelings of anxiety. People are often not highly motivated to get information on cancer. Most people do not like to talk about cancer. These factors do not stimulate people to participate in mass-screening. A significant number of people would even deny symptoms for some time (patient delay). It is therefore not so simple to influence the effectiveness of mass-screening and motivate people to participate by information and health education. Non-participants, however, are sometimes found to belong to the high-risk groups (Wakefield, 1972). Knowledge of the reasons why people do not participate and comparison with participants in mass-screening for cancer may lead us to discover new, more effective ways of informing the non-participants.

To study the effectiveness of mammography as a mass-screening tool we need to know more about the number of participants and non-participants. We also have to obtain more information about their profiles.

NUMBER OF PARTICIPANTS

Except for theoretical reasons there is little need for further research on why women do not participate if the number of women who do participate is relatively high. Unless one expects the number of non-participants to be significantly higher in repeat screenings.

In most studies the percentage of participants is about 65–75, depending on population characteristics such as age, social class, health care system and number of screenings. In the Netherlands, for example, the government considers a 30% drop-out in mass-screening for cervical cancer as 'normal'. In the mammography mass-screening in Nijmegen, which included more than 20 000 women, 85% of the women between 35–65 years took part in the first screening. Given this figure there seems to be no need to investigate the group of non-participants. However, in the first 3 months of the second screening, only 55% showed up; in the age group of 37–65 this constituted 65%. This enormous drop raises the following questions: who are the non-participants and why do they not show up?

WHO IS TAKING PART? WHO IS NOT?

Much research is being done to identify people who are not willing to join preventive screening programmes and to explain why some people delay when they have symptoms. Models have been made to explain this health behaviour and illness behaviour (Kasl and Cobb, 1966; Rosenstock, 1967). It seems the same mechanisms are at work in cases of non-participation and of delay. Summarizing the literature, the factors shown in Table 12.1 seem to be important (van den Heuvel, 1977b).

This summary is not to be considered exhaustive. It is an attempt to sum up the most obvious findings.

RESEARCH TO CHARACTERIZE PARTICIPANTS VERSUS NON-PARTICIPANTS

In the mammography mass-screening at Nijmegen we decided to investigate characteristics of participants versus non-participants. By discovering who they were and why they did or did not participate we hoped to find guidelines for health education which would stimulate people to participate. Based on the literature and within the possibilities of a questionnaire we selected the variables shown in Table 12.2.

Table 12.1

1. Demographic variables		
(a) age	high	non-participants
(b) marital status	unmarried	,,
(c) socio-economic status	low	,,
(d) education	low	,,
2. Personality characteristics		
(a) depressive behaviour	high	non-participants
(b) apathy	high	,,
(c) intellectual capacity	low	,,
(d) inner-directedness	strong	,,
(e) life crises	high	,,
3. Experiences in health care		
(a) consulting doctors	low	non-participants
(b) doctor–patient relationship	bad	,,
(c) trust in medicine	low	,,
4. Social integration		
(a) personal contacts	few	non-participants
(b) family relationship	weak	,,
(c) information by mass media	low	,,
5. Knowledge of disease		
(a) general knowledge of disease	low	non-participants
(b) knowledge of risk factors	low	,,
6. Anxiety		
(a) pain	high	non-participants
(b) death	high	,,
(c) mutilation	high	,,
7. Alienation		
(a) powerlessness	high	non-participants
(b) normlessness (anomia)	high	,,
8. Attitude to prevention		
attitude towards prevention behaviour	negative	non-participants
9. Seriousness of disease		
(a) seriousness	low	non-participants
(b) susceptibility	low	,,

RESEARCH POPULATION AND INTERVIEWS

A representative sample of 195 women who took part in mammography breast screening from early 1975 to June 1976 was prepared. A sample of 222 non-participants was also selected.

In July 1976 these ladies were asked by letter to meet trained female interviewers who tried to collect the data; 140 participants and 82 non-participants cooperated. The interviews lasted $1\frac{1}{2}$ hours each. Reasons for not cooperating are shown in Table 12.3.

The high percentage of wrong addresses of the non-participants (13% versus 7%) and the higher percentage 'not at home' (19% versus 12%) is noticeable. The most important feature among the non-participants however is the number of refusals; three times as high as among participants. (This high number of refusals is always a problem with a retrospective study on this subject. A prospective study is preferable.) Reasons for refusal were:

– no time;
– do not like it;
– not interested in it;
– anxiety through experience of relatives suffering from cancer;
– privacy.

Table 12.2 Concepts and items to differentiate between participants and non-participants

– age	+
– marital status	–
– number of children	–
– education of respondent	–
– occupation of respondent	–
– occupation of husband	+
– house ownership	+
– knowledge of breast cancer (total)	+
– knowledge of symptoms	+
– general knowledge of breast cancer	+
– attitude of denial	+
– perceived seriousness	–
– looking for medical care	+
– delay attitude	–
– normlessness	–
– powerlessness	+
– health anomia	+
– attitude towards prevention	–
– independence ('doing it alone')	+
– asking for advice	–
– talking about illness in neighbourhood	–
– heard about mass-screening in neighbourhood	+
– people in neighbourhood participating in mass-screening	+
– read leaflet on breast cancer	+
– read article in newspaper about breast cancer screening	+
– judgement on information about breast cancer screening	+
– more information wanted on breast cancer screening	+

Table 12.3

	Participants	Non-participants
Wrong address	7%	13%
Not at home (holiday)	12%	19%
Refusals	9%	27%
Others	—	4%
Interviewed	72%	37%
Total	(195)	(222)

ANALYSIS OF VARIANCE

Several items dealing with breast cancer were used to analyse the differences between participants and non-participants. The most important items were reduced by factor-analysis and 'concepts' were constructed based on this factor analysis (van den Heuvel, 1977b). These 'concepts' and items were used to differentiate between participants and non-participants by analysis of variance. In Table 12.2, the results of these analyses of variance are presented; + means the difference between participants and non-participants is significant at least at the 5% level; − means the difference is not significant statistically.

Participants compared with non-participants:

- are younger;
- are in a higher social class by husband's occupation;
- own a house more often;
- have more 'total' knowledge of breast cancer;
- have more knowledge of symptoms of breast cancer;
- have more general knowledge of breast cancer;
- deny cancer less;
- are more frequently attending for medical care;
- have fewer feelings of powerlessness;
- have less health anomia (trust medicine more);
- are less 'independent';
- heard of the mass-screening in the neighbourhood;
- know people in the neighbourhood participating;
- read leaflet;
- react positively to the information provided;
- would like to know more about breast cancer.

These results coincide, in the main, with the findings of other studies. The next questions are:

1. How do these concepts and items relate, interact and relate as a whole to participation?
2. Which are the most important concepts?

STEP-WISE DISCRIMINANT ANALYSIS

To answer the last two questions a step-wise discriminant analysis was used. The step-wise discriminant analysis selects the most important (strongly related) factors where two or more items are strongly related to one another and to participation or non-participation. On this basis the discriminant selects the most significant items to explain who is a participant and who is not. Six concepts were most important when measured by their contribution, for the explanation of participation or non-participation.

The significance of the F value was used to select five items:

Table 12.4

	Standardized discriminant function coefficient
1. People in neighbourhood participating	0.59
2. Attitude of denial	−0.40
3. Read leaflet on breast cancer	0.29
4. Looking for medical care	−0.23
5. Age	0.19

The sixth item was the occupation of the husband, but when measured by the F ratio it was not significant. This item was immediately followed by 'total' knowledge of breast cancer.

Why people do or do not go to mass screening for cancer can be strongly influenced by social integration. The absence of denial of cancer is also important: strong denial (high anxiety) prevents people from going. Not everybody reads the leaflets they get before the screening; written information is not read (and/or understood) by everyone (especially in the lower classes). A person who tends to seek medical attention as soon as the need is felt, is more likely to participate in mass screening. Finally, younger women are more likely to participate than older ones.

The disadvantage of the discriminant analysis is that we do not know which items were eliminated. For example, the standardized discriminant function coefficient of 'total' knowledge of breast cancer is higher than the one of age. Sometimes the 'second best' items may be more useful in the practice of health education.

WHO IS WHO

We have seen that the results of our investigation are in agreement with most research findings. It is certainly possible to 'characterize' participants and non-participants (Table 12.2). Also we may select the most important characteristics.

Do we, however, really know who are participants and who are not? If we think we know – on the basis of these results – we must be able to predict who will participate and who will not, given the characteristics measured. So we asked the computer to classify the individuals according to the five most important characteristics. Without any characteristics one may achieve a score of 63% by classifying everybody as participants (participants – non-participants in our sample: 63% − 37%). With five characteristics the rate of correct prediction was 81%, viz. 91% of the participants and 63% of the non-participants.

QUESTIONS INSTEAD OF CONCLUSIONS

In terms of the whole screened population these last results are disappointing, because in the total population our predictions were 85% correct (percentage of the participants). In the second screening the number of participants dropped significantly, i.e. to 55%.

Of course we have found a number of interesting significant differences between participants and non-participants. The importance of most of these seems to be very small. Do they really tell us who is who?

If we assume that we know who is who, at least in approximately 80% of cases, the question becomes: 'What do we do about it?' How do we reach the non-participants? How do we inform them? How do we decrease the intensity of their denial? How do we supply them with the information they need on the subject of breast cancer? How do we make sure they will read and understand the literature we give them? As for participants, how do we motivate them to come again?

References

Heuvel, W. J. A. van den. (1977a). Image and knowledge of breast cancer of 344 women participating in a mass-screening for breast cancer. Report. Amsterdam (in Dutch)

Heuvel, W. J. A. van den. (1977b). Participants vs. non-participants in mass-screening for breast cancer. Report. Amsterdam (in Dutch)

Kasl, S. and Cobb, S. (1966). Health behavior, illness behavior and sick-role behavior. *In:* Arch. Environmental Health, **12**, pp. 246–266 and 531–541

Rosenstock, I. M. (1966). Why people use health services. *In:* D. Mainland (ed.), Health Services Research, Millbank Memorial Fund Quarterly, **44**

Wakefield, J. (1972). *Seek wisely to prevent.* (London: Her Majesty's Stationery Office)

Discussion

Ray: To explain why people participated or did not participate you looked at demographic and attitudinal variables. Might personality variables have been a better indicator?

van den Heuvel: I think that all these variables are important. We will in further research certainly include personality characteristics as explanatory variables.

Wenderlein: In our experience the rate of drop-out in repeat screening programmes is lowered when the screening procedure goes beyond a simple mammography, when women are also taught self-examination and when they are taught to recognize what is normal and abnormal.

van den Heuvel: In the first screening, participation was as high as it was for a number of reasons: there was much publicity to induce women to participate; the invitation to take part was sent to all women living in one street at a time and women who persuaded one another to go – particularly well-integrated women. Thirdly, women regarded participation as a kind of 'guarantee' against cancer for the next year or so.

When we discovered this last aspect, we adjusted our information accordingly; this partly explains the subsequent decrease in participation. Other factors were less publicity and perhaps the poor follow-up care which was given to those women who had to return for further investigations.

Out of the 20 000 women screened, 240 were invited to attend for further investigations and 70 of these women were found to have cancer. Not all these women were handled well from the psychological point of view and this may have made a bad impression on the other women.

van Brederode: Would it perhaps be important to investigate if non-participants possess the same characteristics as those women who have severe problems after a mastectomy?

van den Heuvel: That would be important. I expect that further research will show that the same explanatory variables are involved in models on health behaviour and on illness behaviour.

General Discussion

Brand: It will of course be impossible to discuss all the aspects of the subject in the time available; so I will have to guide the discussion in such a way that some important aspects, which have not been touched on before, are at least covered. The first aspect: is general information on mammary carcinoma useful?

Maguire: How general should that information be? Do we really want to inform the public at large about survival rates or should we control the information given?

Ray: I think that such information should be controlled. Even the cancer patient is less interested in this sort of detailed information than in how she is doing at present.

van den Heuvel: I disagree with the control of information. It is the patient who should decide what she wants to know and what she does not want to know. The criteria that the medical profession uses to distinguish who should be informed about, for example, diagnosis and prognosis are extremely subjective. Every doctor will tell you that 'it depends' when you ask him if he informs his patients fully, but an American study showed that it does not depend on the patient but on him. Some doctors never inform, others do. The specific situation and circumstances of a particular patient have hardly anything or even nothing to do with the physician's behaviour.

Ray: Yet I believe that if the population is confronted with the fact that such a large percentage are eventually going to die from the disease, even if the diagnosis has been made early, then this discourages women from taking action.

Vermost: It is difficult for the individual to grasp statistical data and to apply these to himself, but it is important that patients learn to discuss such things with their doctor. This will also make patients realize that doctors do not know everything either.

van Keep: I think that oral contraception has already considerably changed the doctor–patient relationship. Women who are on the pill are freer in their relationship with their doctor; they are familiar with the atmosphere in his surgery, the gynaecological examination and the examination of their breasts. For these women the threshold, as far as going to the doctor is concerned, has been lowered by the pill. These women will have fewer problems with participation in screening programmes.

Wenderlein: I agree. The acceptance of screening is part of a learning process that requires many years.

Ray: What degree of explicitness should be considered? I feel that doctors should not avoid the word cancer and should be prepared to volunteer the diagnosis. I do not, however, think that the doctor should spontaneously present the statistics for probability of survival.

Metze: The doctor cannot and should not see his patients as statistics. He never knows exactly on what side of the statistics a particular woman is going to be. He should share his uncertainty with her. My experience is that if he does this the patient can cope better with her problems than if she has received no information at all.

Maguire: I think that it is right to share uncertainty, but I also believe that there should be room for hope. If you leave patients with total uncertainty or without hope they can collapse very easily.

van Keep: Do we all agree that the public should be made aware of the possibility that breast cancer can develop? Should women not be told how great the statistical chances are that they might contract it? It should in any case be explained that an early diagnosis may mean a greater chance of recovery and certainly means a long period of remission during which life can be full of satisfaction.

Gyllensköld: About patient delay: I think that this can be influenced by publicity and education via the mass media. Balanced information may well overcome psychological defence mechanisms.

Maguire: It has been suggested that the behaviour of key members of small communities is of more importance than what the mass media say. Thus it is argued that if the vicar's wife in a small village makes it known that she reacted promptly when she felt a lump in her breast this has more impact than the best programme on TV.

van den Heuvel: You really need both. The mass media should provide the basic information. Mouth-to-mouth information and the behaviour of local 'examples' are, in addition, of paramount importance. The importance of the mass media should be neither over- nor underestimated. The mass media should give people general ideas about disease and about diagnostic and therapeutic possibilities. To ensure, however, that this knowledge is applied, reinforcement by the local community peer groups is needed.

Gyllensköld: I do not think that knowledge as such is lacking. Instead, I think that patient delay can be attributed to feelings of anxiety, fear and mystery. After all, people do not know why they get cancer. They know, or think they know, why many diseases occur: diet, cold, etc., but cancer is a much more mysterious disease. The medical profession reinforces this feeling: as long as doctors avoid the use of the word cancer and as long as doctors are not receptive to the emotions of their patients and of their patients' relatives, cancer will be a mysterious and anxiety-provoking disease.

Ray: Some patients I spoke with were able, years after the mastectomy, to describe their own defensiveness at that time. They told me that they were hiding from themselves the fact that the lump in their breast could be cancer. I am sure that this happens in the case of many women who would never admit to it.

Brand: The doctor himself may be responsible for some of the loss of time occurring between his examination of the lump and the mastectomy: the so-called doctor's delay. What can be done to reduce this?

Gyllensköld: We should not overestimate doctor's delay. It is only responsible for a small fraction of the total delay.

Maguire: The idea of doctor's delay implies that doctors are sometimes deliberately negligent, that they found something that might be cancer but are not referring the patient. I think that the problem is often one of clinical judgement: is a lump likely to be malignant or not? Some clinicians are less skilled and therefore make errors.

Gyllensköld: I am not so certain that it is that simple. The doctor also has psychological defence mechanisms and sometimes he does not see what he does not want to see.

Maguire: Yet I think that few doctors have difficulties in making the diagnosis as such. They become anxious when they have to decide what to tell the patient.

Gyllensköld: Doctors may well need training in this respect: it should be part of the medical curriculum.

van Keep: It must also be a matter of age and maturity. The young doctor, recently qualified, may be pleased to make the right diagnosis but it requires maturity to cope with his own feelings and those of the patient.

Wenderlein: Doctors, young or old, should be trained in empathy. There is no excuse for a doctor who is not able to handle his patient's emotional problems.

Maguire: I do not think you are doing justice to the complexity of medical practice. Maybe the kind of person who is best able to carry out breast cancer surgery at a technical level is less able to talk to his patients about their emotional problems. Indeed, it could be that if he did get involved in that way, he would be less able to make crucial decisions about treatment. What we must demand is that surgeons heed the psychological and social problems involved and enlist the help of other people.

van den Heuvel: I think that you are right. The way to deal with cancer is not only a medico-technical problem but also a social one. It constitutes not only a problem for the patients but also one for the professional helpers.

Brand: Let us move on to the next subject: early detection and the role played by patients and doctors.

van den Heuvel: In Holland there is a current debate on the best methods of carrying out mass-screening. Various possibilities exist such as self-examination, mammography, palpation by professional people or a combination of both mammography and palpation. Should female volunteers be trained to examine other women? Should only the high-risk patients be screened regularly? If so, who are these high-risk patients?

No one knows the answers yet. I think that a case can be made for the encouragement of self-examination, because this method seems fairy effective. On the other hand, there is a distinct disadvantage to mass-screening: people believe that participation in mass-screening serves simultaneously as a kind of protection.

Ray: Another disadvantage of mammography is that the technical equipment which is needed frightens many women. Examination and palpation by others, such as trained volunteers or even medical staff, also has its drawbacks; women are often modest and do not like to undress in front of others and to be touched by others. This applies especially to their breasts. Self-examination will also not be easily accepted by some: a proportion of the population still has inhibitions about touching the breasts.

van den Heuvel: We calculated that if we tried to screen 20 000 women over a period of two years by means of mammography, then about 70% would probably participate. If we tried to convince 20 000 women to carry out a self-examination each month, then we estimated that about 50% would respond. With the first method, with all the expensive technical equipment involved, only eight more cases of cancer would be found than with the second method. We do not even know if the chance of survival of those eight cases would be better or not. It is clear therefore that on the basis of these calculations self-examination is the method of choice for early detection of breast cancer.

Gyllensköld: It has been mentioned before that in more than 70% of all instances of cancer of the breast the lesion was first discovered by the woman herself. One could imagine that mass-screening programmes would have the opposite effect because they remove the woman's own responsibility for her own body. We discovered in Sweden that many teenagers were embarrassed when their breasts began to develop. They flatten their breasts by the use of tight clothing.

We therefore concluded that it would be useful to teach children to get acquainted with their bodies by means of self-palpation in order to try and break this taboo.

van Keep: I have great difficulty in convincing my teen-aged children to brush their teeth because they refuse to understand that if they brush their teeth now they will save on dentists' bills later. How could I convince my daughter at her age that she should develop a type of behaviour now which would be of benefit later on? To me there seems little purpose in telling a young woman, whose breasts are beginning to develop to palpate them now in order to avoid the loss of a breast when she is 50.

Gyllensköld: Learning how to feel a lump is less important than to become fully acquainted with one's own body.

van Keep: Would you, for this purpose, also be in favour of the use of those tactile teaching models that are used to teach students how various types of lumps present on palpation?

Gyllensköld: They could be used and they are of course especially useful for medical students, but I do think that every woman should definitely learn to get used to how her own breasts feel. If a lump developed suddenly, she would realize that a change had occurred which required further investigation.

Humphrey: When should a young girl start learning how her breasts feel, in order to obtain a kind of baseline from which to judge significant changes later?

Gyllensköld: I do not know the answer, but I imagine that she should start between the ages of 12 and 14. Obviously it would be best if this was included in lessons on general hygiene.

Vermost: I think that young girls should be taught to understand their whole bodies rather than just their breasts.

Maguire: I am much in favour of early detection, and want to see its promotion included in teaching and education. But I am still a little worried about indiscriminate heightening of people's awareness that they might have cancer. In some women such campaigns lead to irrational fears and even phobias.

van den Heuvel: There is indeed the tendency for women to become very scared of breast cancer and mastectomy because of all the publicity on these subjects. I think that we should concentrate instead on making public the possibilities of prevention of cancer of the breast and in which ways women can actively participate by means of self-examination. In this way fear and anxiety could be replaced by active participation in prevention and this is what we should aim at.

Brand: The recent publicity on possible harmful and even carcinogenic effects of mammography must have had a great impact on participation. What, moreover, are current opinions on the cost-benefit ratios of screening programmes?

van Keep: Calculation of costs should include psychological costs. Going to the doctor or the screening centre, time spent waiting, undressing and being looked at and palpated by others all add up to quite a psychological 'investment'.

van den Heuvel: Some American investigators have made calculations of costs and benefits. Such calculations are difficult to apply to different countries and, in any case are always easy to criticize.

Brand: When should we regard a woman as being cured? I do of course not refer to the purely medical and oncological point of view but to the point of view of her resignation to the loss of a breast.

Maguire: Ideally every patient should be in direct or indirect – through volunteers – contact with a specially trained nurse. This nurse should be backed up by a team formed at least by a psychiatrist and a social worker. The patient should have access to this team as long as she needs it, however long this may be. The moment of emotional recovery is then determined by the patient herself: when she makes a well-considered decision to terminate contact she has reached the end point of recovery.

Brand: Could anybody make a suggestion on which type of research is needed in the future?

Gyllensköld: I wonder if it would be possible to study the economic aspects of pre-operative counselling. It is known that similar counselling of patients who required elective intra-abdominal operations contributed towards a reduction of their stay in hospital, and of the amount of tranquillizers and sleeping pills they needed after the operation.

Ray: I do not think that you can compare such operations with a mastectomy. Following an abdominal operation there is not the same degree of disfigurement and the patient is also, in general, not left with the same threat to health. I think that in the case of mastectomy patients the emphasis should be on post-operative counselling.

Gyllensköld: I did not exclude the importance of post-operative counselling. I only wanted to draw attention to the fact that more research should be done on the value of pre-operative counselling.

Metze: I would like to see some research done on the best ways in which psycho-social care, in particular of mastectomy patients, could be introduced in those hospitals where physical care is the only criterion of treatment at present.

Maguire: I would be most interested in a transcultural study of the various approaches to psychological intervention. It seems to me that such a study might be very helpful indeed to the approach which each of us uses.

Brand: It seems to me that this last remark makes a perfect ending to our general discussion because it stresses the need for continuing international contact and exchange of views. As far as we are aware, a multinational group such as ours has never before exchanged views on this subject. We, of the International Health Foundation, are of the opinion that this meeting can be called a success if it has made the participants listen to one another's points of view and if it has opened further avenues of research both for us and for others in the future.

Index

Adjustment scores 34, 35, 36, 42
Analysis
    of variants in mass-screening 101
    step-wise discriminant 101
Anxiety scores 42
Anxiety symptoms 48, 50
Axillary lymph nodes 74
Axillary metastases 58

Banks operation 74
Biopsy, breast, anxiety and depression before 48–9
Body cathexis 35, 44
Breast
    anxiety and depression before biopsy 48–9
    delay in different stages of cancer 60
    lump campaign in Stockholm 64
    reconstruction 45, 67–72
        operation techniques for 69–70
    tumourectomies in cancer 76, 77, 79

Cancer
    activism in 94
    early detection 11
    education campaign for 59
    screening programmes for 91–6
    general information on 105
    instrumentalism in 94
Cardiff–St Mary's trial 38
Chemotherapy 55, 79
Cholecystectomy, groups used as controls 34–6, 38, 44
Cobalt radiation 79
Conservative surgery 75, 78

Delay, in different stages of breast cancer 60, 61
'Denial charade' 29
Depressive symptoms 49
Drugs prescribed 51

'Early Cancer Detection Centres' (Belgium) 91

F ratio 102
Freiburg Personality Inventory (FPI-N) 10

Halsted operation 68, 70, 71, 73, 74
Health care, attitudes to 11
Holland, mass-screening in 98, 108
Hormone therapy 79
Husband, confrontation with 27–8

Interviews, after surgical operations 39–40
Introversion–extraversion scale 34, 39

La Fondation Curie (Paris) 75
Liaison nurse scheme 52–3
Lymphoedema 22

Mass-screening 94, 95, 96
    analysis of variants in 101
    effectiveness of 97
    in Holland 98, 108
    number of participants in 98
    variables in 99
Mastectomy 3, 4
    adjustment to 33–43
    body experience in 19
    and the children 29
    comparisons in patients having radio-therapy for 87–8
    as a crisis 28–9
    experiences of women in 15–21
    as a family problem 25–6
    groups 10, 11, 12
    patients' contact with others 19–20
        counsellors for 30
    psychiatric problems after 47–55
    psycho-social adjustment after 9, 11
    radical 83
    reactions after 49–50
    restrictions after 5
Mood disturbance, duration of 50, 52

Nipple reconstruction 71
NISSO (Netherlands Institute for Social-Sexological Research) 15

INDEX

Oncologist, psychological problems of 73–5

Patient
  psychological coping mechanisms in 86–7
  psychological problems of 75–8
Partner, relationship with 20
Personality factors, in mastectomy groups 10–11
Postponing information, in treatment 17–18
Prosthesis 2, 68
Psychiatric problems after mastectomy 47–55
Psychological problems
  of oncologist 73–5
  of patient 75–8
  of surgeon 73–5
Psychological coping mechanisms in patients 86–7
'Psychosomatic illness' 27
Psycho-social adjustment after mastectomy 9, 11

Radiation
  cobalt
  treatment
    concepts of 84–5
    experiences in 85–6
    fears of 84
    questions about 83
Radical mastectomy 83
Radiotherapy 18, 22, 55, 70, 73, 79
  comparisons in patients on, before and after mastectomy 87–8
  psychological coping mechanisms in patients on 86–7
Radiumhummet, Karolinska Sjukhuset, Stockholm 81, 83, 85

Reach to Recovery programme 1–2
  volunteers for 2–3
Reconstruction
  breast 45, 67–72
    operation techniques in 69–70
  nipple 71

Self-examination, best age to start 109
Self-help groups 13
Sexual problems 50–1
Sexual relationship, re-establishing 28, 54
Sociologisch Onderzoeksinstitut (Sociological Research Institute), Stockholm 92
Step-wise discriminant 101–2
Stockholm
  breast lump campaign in 64
  Radiumhummet, Karolinska Sjukhuset 81, 83, 85
  Sociologisch Onderzoeksinstitut (Sociological Research Institute) 92
Surgeon, psychological problems of 73–5
Surgery, conservative 75, 78
Surgical groups, comparison between 38–9

Therapy
  hormone 79
  radiation 83, 84, 85, 86
Treatment
  postponing information in 17–18
  radiation
    concepts of 84–5
    experiences in 85–6
    fears of 84
    questions about 83
Tumourectomies, for breast cancer 76, 77, 79

Vivre comme Avant programme 9

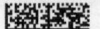